EVALUATION IN A
NUTSHELL

3RD
EDITION

Adrian Bauman | Don Nutbeam

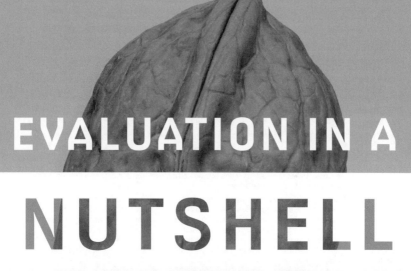

EVALUATION IN A

NUTSHELL

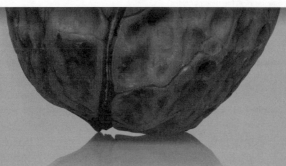

A practical guide to the evaluation
of health promotion programs

McGraw Hill

This Third edition published 2023
First edition published 2006, Second edition published 2014
Text © 2023 Adrian Bauman & Don Nutbeam
Illustrations and design © 2023 McGraw Hill Education (Australia) Pty Ltd

Additional owners of copyright are acknowledged in on-page credits/on the acknowledgments page.
Every effort has been made to trace and acknowledge copyrighted material. The authors and publishers tender their apologies should any infringement have occurred.

National Library of Australia Cataloguing-in-Publication Data:

A catalogue record for this book is available from the National Library of Australia

Authors: Adrian Bauman, Don Nutbeam
Title: Evaluation in a Nutshell: a practical guide to the evaluation of health promotion programs
Edition: 3rd edition

ISBN: 9781760427177

Published in Australia by
McGraw Hill Education (Australia) Pty Ltd
Level 33, 680 George Street, Sydney NSW 2000
Publisher: Rochelle Deighton
Production manager: Martina Vascotto
Copyeditor: Leanne Peters
Proofreader: Meredith Lewin
Permissions manager: Rachel Norton
Cover and internal design: Simon Rattray, Squirt Creative
Cover image: Krzysztof Pazdalski/Shutterstock
Typeset by Straive
Printed in Singapore by Markono Print Media Pte Ltd

contents

CHAPTER 1

Planning for evaluation   1

CHAPTER 2

Research and evaluation in health promotion: key stages, methods and types   17

list of tables and figures

TABLES

Chapter 1

Chapter 2

Chapter 3

Chapter 4

Chapter 5

Chapter 6

FIGURES

Chapter 7

Chapter 8

Chapter 9

about the authors

Adrian Bauman is Emeritus Professor of Public Health and Health Promotion at the University of Sydney, Australia. He directs the World Health Organization (WHO) Collaborating Centre on Physical Activity, Nutrition and Obesity. He has taught health promotion research methods and program evaluation to public health students for 35 years, and is interested in the evaluation methods for scaled-up health promotion programs at the population level.

Don Nutbeam is a Professor of Public Health at the University of Sydney. His career has spanned senior leadership positions in universities, government, health services and international organisations including WHO and the World Bank. He has research interests in the social and behavioural determinants of health, and in the development and evaluation of public health interventions.

Acknowledgements

We would like to acknowledge Dr Karen Lee and Dr Melanie Crane who provided some examples used in this edition of *Evaluation in a Nutshell*.

preface

This book is for students of public health and health promotion and for health promotion practitioners. *Evaluation in a Nutshell* is intended to equip the reader with the ability to understand, interpret and assess the quality of published research, to excite interest in evaluation and promote further study that will lead to the development of core skills in evaluation.

In writing this book, we have drawn on many years of experience in conducting evaluations of health promotion programs, working with practitioners and teaching public health students. From this experience we recognise the need for students and practitioners to understand the basic principles of evaluation in the real-world and the application of these principles in evaluation design, both to conduct evaluations and to assess the work of others.

Any review of published research will reveal that not all health promotion projects, interventions and programs are equally successful in achieving their goals and objectives. Programs are most likely to be successful when the determinants of a health problem are well understood, when the needs and motivations of the target population are addressed and when the context in which the program is being implemented is taken into account. That is, the intervention 'fits' the problem and can contribute to the solution.

Similarly, the evaluation methods for a health promotion program need to fit local priorities and the circumstances of the program. Health promotion and disease prevention has changed over recent decades, both in program content and methods of delivery. Programs can be evaluated in a range of ways, may demand differing levels of resources and may use various evaluation designs. This book illustrates how evaluation questions change as a program evolves and matures. It emphasises that innovative programs need closest scrutiny and comprehensive evaluation. By contrast, interventions that have previously been shown to work in a variety of circumstances, and are low cost and low risk, will require more modest monitoring for accountability and quality control. We identify how the rigorous evaluation of projects with tightly defined objectives in a controlled environment will be different to the evaluation of multi-component and more complex programs, emphasising that no single method or design will be 'right' for all programs.

Evaluation in a Nutshell introduces the practical and scientific challenges in the evaluation of health promotion programs. The book takes a real-life and pragmatic public health perspective. It is not meant to be a comprehensive textbook that includes all methodological aspects of evaluation but provides a guide to real-world methods for assessing programs. Even for experienced researchers and practitioners, the book provides a useful prompt on key issues, as well as guidance on how to organise and conduct evaluation studies.

introduction

Evaluation is the formal process of judging the 'value' of something. In health promotion, an evaluation will determine the extent to which a program has achieved its desired health outcomes. Scientists, health practitioners, politicians and the wider community all have different views on what represents 'value' from a health promotion program, how success should be defined and what should be measured, as shown in the following examples.

- Policymakers and budget managers may judge the success of programs in terms of resource allocation and accountability for these decisions. Success is often defined by the relationship between financial investment and the achievement of health outcomes in the short term.
- Health practitioners need to judge the likely and actual success of a program in achieving its defined health outcomes in real-life situations. Success may be defined in terms of the effectiveness of the program in achieving health outcomes, the practicality of implementation, program sustainability and the maintenance of health gains in the longer term.
- The community that is to benefit from health promotion action may place value on the processes through which a program is conducted, particularly on whether the program is participatory and addresses priorities that the community itself has identified. Success may be defined in terms of relevance to perceived needs and opportunities for community participation.
- Academic researchers judge a program's success (or failure) in order to contribute to the science of and evidence base for health promotion programs and practice. Success may be defined in terms of the effects identified through rigorous scientific evaluation designs and measured through quantifiable and validated outcomes, and where the expected effects are theoretically based.

These perspectives are distinct but not mutually exclusive. In each perspective, success is judged through improved health outcomes, yet each differs greatly in the emphasis given to the cost, practicality and processes involved in achieving these outcomes. Correspondingly, there is a spectrum of approaches used to evaluate health promotion programs. These range from highly structured, methodology-driven evaluations through to much less rigid, highly participatory forms of evaluation.

As public health professionals and practitioners, we need to be accountable for what we do, and we need to make explicit what we expect to achieve through the investments that are made in health promotion and prevention interventions. All programs can benefit from some form of evaluation, but not all require the same intensity of evaluation effort.

This book aims to:

- provide an overview of and a classification system for the evaluation of a health promotion project, program or intervention
- distinguish between formative, process, impact and outcome evaluation
- consider the relative contributions of qualitative and quantitative research methods
- provide practical guidance on when and how to evaluate programs, and the range of evaluation designs and research methods that can be used to evaluate different project and program types
- consider how best to 'measure' health promotion activity and outcomes
- refer the reader to sources of further information.

There is a companion website to accompany this volume, which will be updated regularly by the authors at https://evaluationinanutshell.com/. It is written and maintained by the authors to provide a repository of updated and annotated examples but is not part of this McGraw Hill publication.

1

Planning for evaluation

This chapter introduces the purposes and functions of evaluation and describes the stages in planning and implementing a health promotion or disease prevention program or intervention. These range from defining the problem and developing solutions to planning and implementing programs. Each stage is linked to the evaluation methods described in this book.

Before we start on methods for evaluation, we need to define our terms that describe programs, projects and interventions as we use them throughout the book. These are shown in Table 1.1.

Table 1.1 Projects and programs defined

Term	Our description
Project	A project is a discrete, smaller-scale and well-defined health promotion activity.
Program	Programs are multi-component, usually larger scale health promotion activities, comprised of multiple projects or components; careful consideration of what level of evaluation is needed for each component, and for the whole program of work.
System	System-level activities are health promotion efforts targeting a large-scale whole interconnected system. Evaluation includes the interactions in the system, as well as the effect of the whole systems approach.
Intervention	This is a generic term, widely used in the published scientific literature on health promotion evaluation used to describe health promotion activity at any level or size (usually projects and programs as described above).

Evaluation methods should be considered during the planning stage as an integral part of the development of a project or program. It is far more difficult to 'add' evaluation in at later stages after the critical decisions on program components and implementation have been made.

Successful evaluation of a program is more likely if:

- a thorough population analysis of a health problem will indicate the potential for intervention
- there are clearly defined, logical and achievable program *goals* and *objectives*
- formative assessment is used to develop an intervention, giving sufficient attention to the materials, resources and human capacity required
- the intervention is implemented as planned and a good record of the implementation is kept
- the project or program is of sufficient size, duration and sophistication to be able to demonstrate if it is effective or ineffective in relation to its goals and objectives
- there is a clear plan for implementing the evaluation
- the evaluation provides sufficient relevant information to those deciding the program's value.

Achieving these conditions for successful evaluation is challenging, but more likely if a structured approach to planning is adopted.

Planning models are commonly used in the development and management of health promotion programs. Such models support evidence-led practice and provide a foundation for program evaluation. Some models of planning use population-level and individual enablers, facilitators and barriers to identify the best approach to project planning (Green & Kreuter 2022); others use planning models to specify the intervention components to be delivered.

Using a planning model enables a logical sequence of considering the likelihood of achieving the program goals and objectives through each step and strategy planned for the program. A planning model provides a structured description of how the impacts of, and outcomes from, a health promotion intervention develop over time and also provides a sound foundation for the evaluation of an intervention (see Chapter 3).

Figure 1.1 presents the health promotion planning and evaluation 'cycle' related to that used in the companion volume to this book, *Theory in a Nutshell: A Practical Guide to Health Promotion Theories* (Nutbeam et al. 2022). This describes the various stages in planning, implementing and evaluating a health promotion program. In this chapter, we consider each of these stages in turn, focusing on the evaluation tasks and methods at each stage.

Figure 1.1 The planning and evaluation cycle

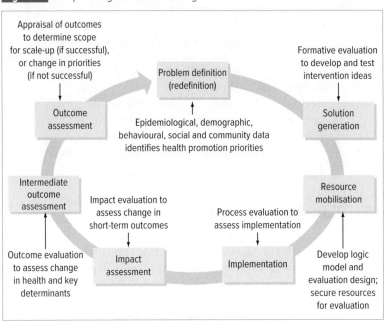

1.1   Problem definition: starting at the end

A wide range of information can be used to define a health problem and generate potentially effective solutions. This may include routinely collected epidemiological, demographic, behavioural and social information, and can be enhanced by local community needs assessments. At this *information-gathering* stage, it is important to consider the following.

- What is the overall size (prevalence) of the problem? How many people in the target population are likely to be affected by the problem?
- How prevalent is the problem in various subgroups (e.g. older adults, adolescents or people from socially disadvantaged or culturally diverse populations)?
- What is the strength of the relationship between the problem and health outcomes? How serious is the problem for the individuals affected and the population as a whole (e.g. does it contribute to disability, reduced quality of life or reduced mental health, and does it increase health service usage or increase costs or contribute to premature death)?

- Does the problem have any impact outside health (e.g. environmental, economic or other sectors)?
- What is the potential for intervention? Can some factors or conditions be realistically influenced that will have an impact on the problem (these may be behavioural, social or environmental, or relate to improved health services)? Does it fit with current government or national priorities for action?
- What evidence is there that this intervention has the capacity to produce the desired improvements in risks or conditions and improve public health?
- What evidence is there that the community recognises the problem and gives priority to addressing it?

1.2 Planning a solution

The second stage in the cycle prompts analysis of potential solutions, leading to the development of a *program/project plan* that specifies the intervention components. Planning for a whole program of work is more complex and multifaceted than planning for a more limited individual project, because it involves clearer sequencing and the use of a wider range of measures for success. These differences between projects and program evaluation are discussed in greater detail throughout this book.

This stage in the planning process indicates how and when change might be achieved in the target population, organisation or policy. The planning process leads to the selection of effective interventions that might achieve change and planning the timing and sequencing of interventions designed to achieve maximum effect. This stage in the planning process can be supported by techniques such as *intervention mapping* (IM) and *logic models.* These describe how the project or program elements are expected to work, involving a structured description of what will happen during a program and what changes the project or program intends to bring about and with what anticipated effects. These planning processes and techniques can be greatly supported by *formative evaluation* (before a program is launched), described in Chapter 3.

A theoretical framework or model often underpins the planning of health promotion programs, guiding the project or program's content. These theories can be considered using a socioecological framework and may include strategies to influence individuals, small groups and/or communities, environments and policies. Further information on theories and models in health promotion practice can be found in Nutbeam, Harris & Wise (2022). A range of potential intervention methods can be used. For example, a discrete project using a single intervention method (such as education) in a well-defined setting (such as a school) may make detailed use of individual behaviour change theory, and the evaluation process and outcomes will usually be relatively easy to define and measure. In a more comprehensive program that uses multiple intervention strategies in different settings and targeting different populations, the task of evaluation is inevitably more complex and contestable. The interdependence of the various health promotion actions can make it difficult to assess their individual contributions to outcomes and poses challenges in choosing evaluation methods and analysing results. These challenges in *evaluation design* and the differences between evaluating *projects* and *programs* are considered more fully in Chapters 5 and 6.

Program strategies that incorporate the right combination of actions in the right sequence completes the planning stage of the program and should link clearly and logically to the project or program outcomes. Some modification of the *objectives* may be required at this stage, together with refinements to the *measures* used to evaluate a program's short-term impact.

It is essential to define the sequencing of the intervention in this second step of the planning process. This is evaluated though assessing the project or program implementation that has led to progress (or lack of progress) in achieving program goals and objectives. This is described in more detail in Chapter 4.

1.3 Creating the right conditions for the successful implementation of programs

This stage of program planning (stage 3 in Figure 1.1) is concerned with obtaining the resources (e.g. money, staff and materials) required for successful implementation. In addition, it is concerned with building capacity in a community or organisation to enable an intervention to be introduced and sustained, and to generate the community and political support necessary for successful implementation.

In some circumstances, the resource assessment or the formative evaluation of methods and materials may show that the available resources or community response do not match what is needed. This is also known as 'evaluability assessment', assessing whether the program will deliver on intended goals and objectives and is ready for evaluation. Where there is a mismatch, it may be necessary to reformulate the program to better fit available resources or to generate additional resources and opportunities for action. This planning stage is important whether the intervention is a simple, time-limited project or a more complex, long-term program with multiple components.

Insufficient attention to this phase in the development of a program, including the pre-testing of methods and materials, is a common reason for program failure. This is especially true when program delivery involves working through partners, such as schools, worksites and different government agencies.

1.4   Implementation of health promotion projects and programs

The next stage in the cycle is implementation (stage 4 in Figure 1.1, and Chapter 4). The aim is to ensure that a program will be delivered as closely as possible to the original plan, recognising that implementation in 'real-life' conditions will often require adaptation. Collecting information on program implementation is important at this stage. This *process evaluation* will enable examination of program *fidelity* (the extent to which a program was implemented as planned) and the relationship between implementation and subsequent outcomes.

There may be pressure to implement projects with insufficient resources, within time frames that are too short or in communities that are not ready for the intervention. Such pressure often leads to incomplete project implementation and may produce insufficient evidence on the program's *effectiveness*.

Traditionally, health promotion interventions have emphasised methods designed to promote individual behaviour change. Increasingly, health promotion programs are designed to influence the social, environmental and economic factors that determine health. This requires working through professional groups and directly with communities to mobilise social action and to advocate for political and organisational change. Combining the delivery of different interventions and securing the necessary partnerships to achieve desired *health promotion outcomes* are challenges for practitioners at this stage in more comprehensive programs.

1.5   Health promotion actions and outcomes

It is important to specify a range of measurable (and reliable and valid) *outcomes* in the program plan. These outcomes range from the direct 'impact' of health promotion activities in the short term to *health outcomes* in the longer term. These levels of program effects are shown in Figure 1.1 as stages 5 to 7. They provide an overview of the relationship between the 'processes' of health promotion and the different types of impact and outcome that such interventions might produce.

A comprehensive health promotion program (see Chapter 6) might consist of multiple interventions targeted at different types of outcomes. A shorter term project might focus on achieving a smaller subset of health promotion outcomes. Figure 1.2 shows a typology that characterises these different health promotion actions and the subsequent measures that can be used to assess their impact and outcomes.

Working from the end points on the right-hand side of the model in Figure 1.2, *health and social outcomes* reflect the eventual end points of health promotion and preventive interventions. Thus, outcomes such as quality of life, functional independence and equity have the highest value in the model. Some health outcomes are more narrowly defined in terms of disease outcomes and physical and mental health status. For example, for an HIV-prevention program, the primary health outcome would be to reduce HIV infection rates and AIDS-related mortality.

Intermediate health outcomes represent the *determinants* (immediate and likely causes) of health and social outcomes. Behavioural determinants provide protection from disease or injury (such as physical activity) or increase risk of ill health (such as tobacco use) and are represented as *healthy lifestyles* in the model. The physical environment can reduce people's access to facilities or represent a direct hazard to their physical safety, and economic and social conditions can enhance or limit people's ability to adopt recommended behaviours. These determinants are represented as *healthy environments*. Access to, and appropriate use of, preventive services are acknowledged as an important determinant of health status and are represented as *effective preventive health services*.

For example, a multi-component program designed to reduce COVID-19 infection rates in the long term might have a *project* component targeted at marginalised, disadvantaged populations. In this case, the project might be directed towards:

- achieving preventive behaviours (social distancing, mask wearing) among the target populations
- delivery systems that provide affordable access to COVID-19 testing, vaccination and new proven therapies for the target population.

At the previous stage, *health promotion outcomes* (Figure 1.2) refer to modifiable personal, social and environmental factors that lead to the determinants of health (intermediate health outcomes). These may represent the immediate results of planned health promotion activities. Thus, they include measures of the cognitive and social skills that determine the ability of individuals to gain access to, understand and use health information

Figure 1.2 Health promotion actions and outcomes

Health promotion actions	Health promotion outcomes (outcomes of the process of intervention)	Intermediate health outcomes (program impact, or short-term outcomes)	Social health outcomes (long-term outcomes)
Education Examples include patient education, school education and broadcast media communication	*Health literacy* Measures include health-related knowledge, attitude, motivation, behavioural intentions, personal skills and self-efficacy	*Healthy lifestyles* Measures include tobacco use, physical activity, food choices and alcohol and illicit drug use	*Social outcomes* Measures include quality of life, functional independence, social capital and equity
Social mobilisation Examples include community development, group facilitation and technical advice	*Social action and influence* Measures include community participation, community empowerment, social norms and public opinion	*Effective preventive health services* Measures include access to and provision of relevant and preventive services	
Advocacy Examples include lobbying, political organisation and activism, and overcoming bureaucratic inertia	*Healthy public policy and organisational practices* Measures include policy statements, legislation, regulation and resource allocation organisational practices	*Healthy environments* Measures include safe physical environment, supportive economic and social conditions, good food supply and restricted access to tobacco/alcohol	*Health outcomes* Measures include reduced morbidity, reduced disability and avoidable mortality

(*health literacy* in the model). For example, health literacy comprises health knowledge and an understanding of how to access health and support services. *Social action and influence* comprise organised efforts to promote or enhance the actions and control by social groups over the determinants of health. This includes social mobilisation and securing the resources to overcome structural barriers to health, enhance social support and reinforce social norms conducive to health. Examples of outcomes range from improved social 'connectedness' and social support to improved community empowerment.

Healthy environments are largely determined by *healthy public policy and organisational practices.* Policy-driven legislation, funding, regulations and incentives may significantly influence organisational practices. Thus, examples of health promotion outcomes might be changes to health and social policies that lead to improvements in services, social benefits, the built environment and housing. These would influence organisational practices and redirect resource allocation to support environments conducive to health.

Using the COVID-19 prevention program as an example, health promotion outcomes could include:

■ improving health literacy by raising community awareness regarding COVID-19 prevention and improving skills in accessing trustworthy information on COVID-19 testing or immunisation

■ facilitating a supportive environment through social action, policies and services to improve the delivery systems for COVID-19 testing and treatments and to support other evidence-based preventive behaviours; this may be particularly relevant for higher risk populations (e.g. older adults in residential care, frontline health workers, young children).

Figure 1.2 also indicates three health promotion actions—what to do, as distinct from what outcomes are achieved. The evaluation task is to assess the implementation of these actions. *Education* aims to raise levels of personal health literacy and thereby increase the capacity of individuals and communities to act to improve and protect their health. *Social mobilisation* is action taken in partnership with individuals or social groups to mobilise social and material resources for health. *Advocacy* is action taken on behalf of individuals and/or communities to overcome structural barriers to the achievement of health.

In the example of COVID-19 prevention, these health promotion actions could include:

■ tailored COVID-19 communications using appropriate media to reach diverse communities

■ engaging local community and faith leaders in community mobilisation to encourage COVID-19 vaccination uptake

- local advocacy to improve health service delivery systems and train health professionals to meet the needs of diverse local communities.

Another example of this hierarchy of actions and outcomes can be considered for preventing e-cigarette use among teenagers. Social and health outcomes include reduced incidence of tobacco smoking, and thereby reduced tobacco-related morbidity and mortality, but these outcomes may occur decades after the original program. Intermediate outcomes include reduced e-cigarette use and reduced conversion to tobacco smoking. Health promotion outcomes would include measures of intention to not smoke or use e-cigarettes, changes to social and peer norms and implementation of policies restricting e-cigarette advertising or purchases. In the first column of Figure 1.2, *health promotion actions* in this example would comprise: *education* of young people; *social mobilisation* of parents and other social role models to make e-smoking less attractive and acceptable to young people; and *advocacy* for legislative action to reduce advertising of and access to e-cigarettes.

Figure 1.2 can be used to illustrate not only the links *between* different levels of outcomes but also those *within* levels. For example, among the intermediate outcomes, *action to create healthy environments* may be a direct determinant of social and health outcomes (e.g. by producing a safe working and living environment or improving equity in access to resources), and also separately influence healthy lifestyles (e.g. by reducing access to tobacco products). There is a dynamic relationship between these different outcomes and the three health promotion actions; it is not the static, linear relationship that the model in Figure 1.2 might suggest.

By starting this way, the planning and evaluation process is firmly focused on the end-point outcomes and identifies shorter term measures that are logically related to their achievement. This phase ensures that there is a clear definition of the target of the intervention (subpopulation group, environmental or organisational element) and what outcomes need to be measured. The principles of measurement are described further in Chapter 5.

1.6 Evaluation

Different evaluation tasks occur at each stage of the cycle shown in Figure 1.1. These start with *formative evaluation,* to develop and pre-test program materials and methods (see Chapter 3), and *process evaluation,* to assess program implementation (see Chapter 4).

Health promotion interventions have different types of *impact* and different *outcomes* over time. Change in the outcomes will appear according to different program timescales, depending on the nature of the intervention and the type of social or health problem being addressed. As a consequence, different evaluation methods and measures are needed at different stages in the life of a program.

Impact evaluation measures the short-term effects predicted and defined during the planning stage of the program. These health promotion outcomes (Figure 1.2) are intended to lead to subsequent change in *intermediate health outcomes* (e.g. in behaviours and environments) in ways that will ultimately improve health and social outcomes. Outcome assessment is the end point of health promotion programs and involves improvements in health or changes to the social, economic and environmental conditions that determine health (Figure 1.2).

Figure 1.3 illustrates how a comprehensive set of health promotion interventions might produce different outcomes over time. This model was originally developed to illustrate likely progress over a 5-year period in a comprehensive, community-based, heart disease prevention program. The 'units of time' are years, and this model shows that after 1 year, the program could be measured in terms of increased community awareness and participation. By the 3rd year, progress in health promotion outcomes should be measurable, and after 5 years major progress in intermediate health outcomes should be observable. This model needs to be customised for each program, and to estimate the feasible timescales required to achieve different levels of impact and outcome to funders and decision-makers. This can be invaluable in managing expectations and promoting fairness in accountability for success over time.

Figure 1.3 Theoretical distribution over time of outcomes from health promotion interventions

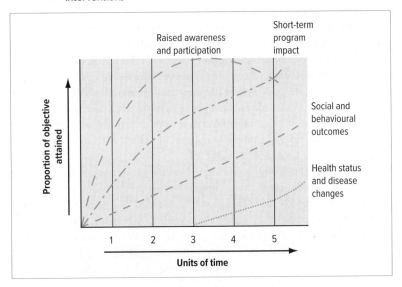

The model in Figure 1.3 will vary according to the type and intensity of intervention. For example, a public education project to promote uptake of a new childhood vaccine may achieve rapid progress in raising awareness, achieving behaviour change (a simple, one-off action is required) and health outcomes (rapid reduction in the population incidence of vaccine-preventable disease). Similarly, a successful smoking-cessation intervention for pregnant women or a fall-prevention trial among the elderly may rapidly demonstrate health outcomes in terms of improved infant birth weight or reduced injuries in older people, respectively. In these examples, the 'units of time' may be months, not years.

Practitioners and evaluators are often faced with unreasonable expectations from impatient policymakers and funders. Explaining the complexity of interventions and the time lag expected between intervention and observable effects can be a challenging task for evaluators.

1.7 Summary

The planning and evaluation cycle (Figure 1.1) illustrates the different stages and their relationships in the development of a plan of action, implementation of the plan and evaluation of outcomes. These processes lead either to successful outcomes that can be considered for further dissemination and scale-up (see Chapter 7) or, if not successful in achieving the intended outcomes, to a re-definition of the proposed solutions—hence to a 'cycle' of planning and evaluation. Because there are several stages, and often a long delay between implementation and outcome, it is often difficult to demonstrate a causal relationship between health promotion actions and long-term outcomes, so it is essential that relevant and appropriate measures are used to clearly measure progress at each stage. A systematic approach to planning and using tools such as *logic models* or *intervention maps* help to anticipate some of these complexities, identify relevant indicators for evaluation and support effective communication and expectation management. The use of logic models in program planning is described in Box 1.1.

The cycle summarised in Figure 1.1 will not address all the issues in planning a health promotion program—real-life decision-making never follows such a smooth path. This model is intended as a guide to be adapted to prevailing circumstances rather than adopted wholesale without critical examination of its usefulness. Few programs have the resources to apply this model in the comprehensive way described here. For these reasons, systematic planning identifies what is possible, makes explicit the program's likely impact and outcomes, and indicates alternative ways to strengthen the intervention. The outcomes illustrated in Figure 1.3 can help define realistic timescales to key stakeholders and can form a basis for periodic program review and accountability. The explicit communication of these limitations also helps to set realistic public and political expectations.

> *In order to plan and perform a high-quality evaluation, it is important to consider the limitations of what each program can achieve in a range of circumstances.*

BOX 1.1: Logic models: a method of summarising a program plan

A *logic model* is a summary depiction of program inputs (human, financial and material resources), the context of the program (factors that may influence the implementation and impact of the intervention) and the activities that together make up the intervention (program events, groups, training, social marketing and so on). A logic model then describes how these intervention elements and activities might result in health promotion outcomes as well as intermediate and end-point outcomes.

In the planning process, a logic model is a 'live' statement, capable of modification over time in response to changed circumstances and available resources. The logic model should, whenever feasible, be actively co-developed by policymakers or practitioners and with community members or stakeholders. The logic model is the final part of the planning phase, describing the project or program's conceptual framework and anticipated effects. If any stage is seen as unachievable or unrealistic, then adjustments to the model can occur before that set of activities is implemented.

An example of a logic model for health promotion is shown in Table 1.2. The logic model shown describes a hypothetical program with the goal of improving healthy food sold in school canteens in a region or school district. The stages in the logic model describe the *program inputs, health promotion actions, health promotion outcomes, intermediate health outcomes* (impact evaluation), and *health and social outcomes*. The planning process describes the anticipated changes for each stage of the logic model. For example: curriculum and resource development are indicators of success in health promotion actions; the implementation of education programs and distribution of resources are health promotion outcomes; and changes in behaviour by students are among the indicators of impact of the program. Mapping these levels of proposed change as part of the pre-intervention planning provides a detailed set of evaluation indicators to be developed.

Table 1.2 Hypothetical logic model: planning a health promotion program to improve healthy food in school canteens

Resources and inputs	Delivery of intervention: state education department/school councils or boards; local public health department (health promotion practitioners); school parent and teacher groups			
Activities	**Education**	**Communication**	**Organisational development**	**Intersectoral/ policy development**
Inputs	Teacher time; parents; canteen managers and suppliers	Teachers, parent and teacher committees; marketing professionals; media chosen	Planning meetings; formation of a steering group; garnering resources	Within-school re-orientation to health and nutrition as priority issues; reach out to parents; food suppliers
Activities (health promotion actions)	Writing of best-practice curriculum for 'healthy eating' among teenagers	Development of media resources (formative testing with students); campaign materials for school canteens	Planning meetings held; partnership developed; planning/ logic model developed	School council/ board makes policy changes regarding healthy nutrition offered in canteens
Outputs (health promotion outcomes)	Education programs implemented; staff and students aware of program	Resources in all canteens; teachers aware of and accept program	Healthy choices approved for canteens; budget and financial model approved	Steering group works towards implementing policy for healthy canteen choices in schools

Resources and inputs	Delivery of intervention: state education department/school councils or boards; local public health department (health promotion practitioners); school parent and teacher groups			
Activities	Education	Communication	Organisational development	Intersectoral/ policy development
Intermediate health outcomes (impact evaluation)	Attempts at behaviour change; healthy eating choices increased among students	Parents and teachers have more favourable views of program; parents' advocacy for program increases	Working groups influence local food environment in schools	Policies around healthy food choices adopted in schools
Health and social outcomes	Reduced obesity and cardiovascular risk among children	Increased sense of school community generalises to other school issues	Health promotion and education work together around other issues	Sustained healthy food choices due to widespread policy adoption

A related concept is *intervention mapping (IM)* which combines formative planning with behavioural theory. There are six stages in IM, starting with: 1. problem analysis and logic models, followed by 2. models of and objectives for change, 3. identifying feasible theories and evidence-based behaviour-change programs, 4. designing the overall program, 5. developing strategies for reach and implementation, and 6. having an overall process and outcome evaluation plan (Fernandez et al. 2019).

References

Fernandez ME, Ruiter RAC, Markham CM, et al. (2019). Intervention mapping: theory- and evidence-based health promotion program planning: perspective and examples. Frontiers in Public Health 7(Aug):209.

Green LW & Kreuter MW (2022). Health Program Planning: An Educational and Ecological Approach, 5th edn. McGraw-Hill, New York, NY.

Nutbeam D, Harris E & Wise M (2022). Theory in a Nutshell: A Practical Guide to Health Promotion Theories, 4th edn. McGraw-Hill, Sydney.

Case studies (abstracts) are annotated and updated in detail on the companion Evaluation website: https://evaluationinanutshell.com/.

Further reading

Community Research (n.d.). Logic models and theory of change. What works New Zealand. The Tangate Whenua, Community and Voluntary Sector Research Centre. Online: https://whatworks.org.nz/logic-model/.

De-Regil LM, Peña-Rosas JP, Flores-Ayala R, et al. (2014). Development and use of the generic WHO/CDC logic model for vitamin and mineral interventions in public health programmes. Public Health Nutrition 17(3):634-9.

Donaldson A, Lloyd DG, Gabbe BJ, et al. (2017). We have the programme, what next? Planning the implementation of an injury prevention programme. Injury Prevention 23(4):273-80.

Lamort-Bouché M, Sarnin P, Kok G, et al. (2018). Interventions developed with the Intervention Mapping protocol in the field of cancer: a systematic review. Psycho-Oncology 27(4):1138-49.

Mills T, Lawton R & Sheard L (2019). Advancing complexity science in healthcare research: the logic of logic models. BMC Medical Research Methodology 19(1):1-11.

Naimoli JF, Frymus DE, Wuliji T, et al. (2014). A community health worker 'logic model': towards a theory of enhanced performance in low- and middle-income countries. Human Resources for Health 12(1):1-16.

Reed MS, Bryce R & MacHen R (2018). Pathways to policy impact: a new approach for planning and evidencing research impact. Evidence and Policy 14(3):431-58.

2

Research and evaluation in health promotion: key stages, methods and types

This chapter provides an overview of the different research methods that support the planning process described in Chapter 1. In particular, the chapter describes differences between research- and practice-based evaluation and explains the use of both quantitative and qualitative methods in evaluation. It summarises the six key stages of evaluation required to build an evidence base for health promotion and public health programs. These different approaches are described in greater detail in later chapters.

Evaluation is not a single action but a set of continuous tasks that start in the planning phase and continue throughout effectiveness testing and subsequent translation of an *intervention,* project or program. This chapter describes these stages of evaluation applied to health promotion and public health interventions.

2.1 Evaluation methods and types

Health promotion projects and programs vary in scope, scale, target population and setting. Four hypothetical examples are described below, and illustrate the differences in the evaluation tasks required.

1. A single project encouraging people attending a regional diabetes clinic to build skills that enable improved control over their disease and its effects and adopting healthier lifestyles
2. A project that aims to increase attendance by an underserved population at a regional cancer screening clinic (e.g. women from a culturally diverse background may have lower screening attendance rates)
3. A program promoting healthy eating in a community in a defined region, comprised of several intervention components, including mass media education, nutrition education in school classrooms and a project to introduce healthy menu choices in restaurants, schools and worksites across the community
4. A multiple-agency partnership between urban planning and transport departments aiming to use new urban designs for housing and

recreational facilities to achieve improvements in the whole system—
improving the physical and social environment to increase physical
activity and wellbeing in the community

There is a distinction between the first two projects, which are discrete
and have clear components, and examples three and four, which are more
complex and comprehensive interventions. The evaluation methods and
measures of outcome required are substantially different. In the first two, the
target population is well-defined and the intervention is quite self-contained,
suggesting well-controlled evaluation studies are possible (Chapter 5).
The second two examples have multiple intervention components and
considerable dependence on partnership with and between agencies and
sectors. The evaluation methods required for these programs are discussed in
Chapter 6, as comprehensive program evaluations (CPEs).

It is obvious from these four examples that there is no single, correct
approach to evaluation. Interventions exist on a continuum, from single-
component through to comprehensive multi-component programs. Evaluation
of the four examples will differ in terms of the budgets required, length of
time required for evaluation, evaluation designs and research methods used.
Customised approaches should be used to plan, implement and evaluate each
project or program.

The first example is set in a health facility and will involve a small (selected)
number of individuals receiving a high level of support to develop the skills
necessary to manage their condition. Key evaluation challenges here will
include research design and measurement. Assessing changes in skills and
self-management practices (e.g. self-efficacy and successful chronic
disease self-management practices) will need to be measured. This evaluation
may compare change in those that participate in the intervention population with
a control group who do not receive the intervention. Such a scientific research
design will allow for a full assessment of the project's *efficacy*—evaluating the
intervention under controlled or 'best possible' conditions.

The second example is a project in a multicultural community-based
setting, and its success and sustainability will depend on the engagement
of community stakeholders and the target population. The evaluation will
consider how well the health promotion workers engage with the community,
and how well the cancer screening service is delivered to this community. The
outcome is increased attendance and screening rates among this community
over time. Such a project may be less amenable to rigorous assessment of
efficacy, but more likely to provide evidence of *effectiveness;* that is, the extent
to which a health promotion intervention is successful in 'real-life' conditions.

The third example is a community-wide program that will include
engagement with different stakeholders in schools, worksites and restaurants;

negotiation will be required to define program goals and objectives, and assess how well an optimal program, given available resources, can be delivered to the participating organisations. The outcomes will include availability of healthy food choices in various settings, including canteens, vending machines and restaurants, and changes in the food choices made by those using these facilities. Assessing the mass media component of the program may involve community surveys to assess changes in awareness and knowledge of healthy eating. An equity perspective for this evaluation might consider whether the intervention reached and influenced different groups across the community.

The fourth example is an intersectoral systems-level program. Assessing the common program needs across agencies is an important first step, followed by an assessment of how well the agencies can partner together towards a common task. In this case the challenge is to build health-promoting environments over a number of years. The outcomes may include coalition-building across agencies, changes to urban and built environment policies, implementation of those policies and assessment of such changes on physical activity participation or community wellbeing.

2.2 Balancing scientific design with practical need

Chapter 1 notes that the concepts of *relevance, efficacy* and *effectiveness* will vary among research scientists, practitioners, policymakers and community members. Researchers value optimal scientific designs that provide evidence through scientific methods and academic publication of results. These evaluations seek to provide evidence of *efficacy,* showing that a project *can* work under optimal conditions, with dedicated staff delivering the program to a motivated study population. This may provide good-quality (best case) evidence that the program can work, but such evidence may not be generalisable or transferable to the wider community. For example, a project that produced good results under 'optimal' conditions with a motivated and engaged population might not produce the same effects if conducted in a poorer neighbourhood with diverse cultural groups, or delivered by busy health practitioners in everyday real-life conditions.

By contrast, when community stakeholders and practitioners manage an evaluation, its design is often more flexible and adaptive, reflecting the less predictable course of many community interventions and the need to adapt to changing circumstances. *Co-creation* is often used here, a process of community partnerships between researchers or other stakeholders in the design, delivery and sometimes evaluation of health promotion programs. This approach may produce information that practitioners value and answer questions about the project's usefulness and relevance to its participants. This type of evaluation may be less likely to produce convincing 'scientific' evidence that any change was directly 'caused' by the intervention (*internal validity*), but can provide compelling evidence on the *external validity* or *generalisability* of an intervention.

Table 2.1 summarises key differences between the perspectives of researchers and practitioners. For the purposes of illustration, it provides a slightly exaggerated view of these differences in perspective, and there is no suggestion that those interested in advancing scientific understanding are not interested in health promotion practice, or vice versa.

> What will become apparent through an examination of the elements in Table 2.1 is that both science and practice are co-dependent, and are best served by a 'middle way': an integrated approach that involves an evaluation partnership meeting both researcher and practitioner needs.

Such an approach will focus attention on not only the practicality and relevance of an intervention for a specific population, but also the scientific value of a program, and supports collaboration between researcher and practitioner to this end.

Table 2.1 The differences and similarities between practitioner and scientific perspectives of health promotion programs

Function	Practitioner perspective (informs program implementation)	Scientific perspective (provides scientific levels of evidence)
Control of program, resources	Controlled by managers and/or stakeholders; evaluation carried out for accountability to funding agencies; practice-led evaluation	Researcher/academic investigator-led evaluation; may be externally funded by scientific grants; research goals of furthering knowledge, academic publication
Purpose of evaluation (accountability)	Identify 'effectiveness' in real-world conditions; used to implement and improve programs, not to 'prove' that programs work; provides evidence on the need for more or different allocation of resources	Aim to generate scientific evidence of program 'efficacy'; can the project or program work in optimal controlled research conditions

Function	Practitioner perspective (informs program implementation)	Scientific perspective (provides scientific levels of evidence)
Research methods	*Quantitative* and *qualitative methods; realist evaluation;* mixed methods; *triangulate* results from different perspectives Apply pragmatic mix of evaluation methods based on needs and/or funding Conclusions may include qualitative judgments of practitioners or the community	Usually evidence from quantitative methods; emphasis on optimising research designs, *statistical significance;* conclusions flow logically from results Attention to methodological issues such as selection *bias* (who participates), measurement *reliability* and *validity;* control for confounding
Level of evaluation	Emphasis on formative evaluation, community consultation, needs assessments Emphasis on process evaluation—monitoring how well activities are implemented and delivered; may adapt program in response to process evaluation findings	Strong emphasis on impact and outcome evaluation and providing 'proof' or evidence of program effects; attention to adherence to the research protocol (*fidelity*)
Research design	Flexible and pragmatic program design to fit the context and target groups addressed by the program	Controlled research designs, with greater measurable focus; may have single outcomes and shorter time frames to assess outcomes
Single focus versus comprehensive approach	Often multi-component programs, with partnerships and interagency collaboration usual; duration—several years with interventions at multiple levels	May be single component for interventions in a specific group; often theory or framework based; follow-up usually short term, typically effects measured between 3 and 12 months

(Continued)

Table 2.1 *Continued*

Function	Practitioner perspective (informs program implementation)	Scientific perspective (provides scientific levels of evidence)
Uses of results	Program failure leads to program improvement and modification; program failure may disappoint decision-makers or the community such that support is withdrawn Successful programs lead policymakers to consider efforts at *scaling-up* (dissemination) more widely to get the program used and adopted in other communities or settings	Contributes to scientific pool of evidence around the efficacy of this type of intervention Successful programs may need *replication* in different settings to examine if similar effects are produced Interventions that show repeated success are amenable to (1) systematic review or *meta-analysis* to summarise results and (2) implementation research to test best methods of reaching more people

Partnerships between funding agencies, researchers, practitioners, communities, stakeholders or participants improve the breadth and relevance of the evidence available from programs. Health promotion science and practice can only advance if we first know whether interventions can work in optimal conditions, and then how and why they work and whether they meet the needs of communities and stakeholders. Each element is important; concentrating on one to the exclusion of others will make what is found less useful.

2.3 Stages of evaluation

Figure 2.1 provides the core evaluation framework for this book. It shows the research and evaluation questions that are addressed stage by stage in the planning and evaluation of health promotion projects and programs. Additional components to this model are added in considering scale-up in Chapter 7. Brief definitions of the types of evaluation are shown in Box 2.1.

The early stages relate to the development and testing of an intervention, while later stages are concerned with the scale-up and adoption of effective

BOX 2.1: The three key types of health promotion evaluation

- *Formative evaluation:* activities designed to develop and pre-test project or program materials and methods, directed towards answering questions concerning relevance to identified health problems and the feasibility of different intervention methods (see Chapter 3).
- *Process evaluation:* activities directed towards assessing progress in project/program implementation and recording the extent to which the program was delivered as planned and the circumstances in which it could be successfully and routinely reproduced (see Chapter 4).
- *Impact (or outcome) evaluation:* measures the effects that are expected to occur as a result of the program.

individual interventions. Stages 1 and 2 indicate the different forms of background descriptive research to understand the problem, profile the target population and develop an intervention plan, as well as *formative evaluation* to test the proposed program components (see Chapter 3 for more detail).

Stage 3 represents the optimal evaluation of a relatively discrete individual project or a more complex program to answer questions of efficacy (can it work) and effectiveness (real-world effects) (see Chapter 5). This includes *process evaluation,* and assessment of the *impact and outcome* of the individual program. This type of study helps make decisions about whether the intervention warrants further testing and wider dissemination.

At stage 4, the intervention is replicated and tested in other settings to assess whether or not it works as well in other settings; this is a necessary precursor to scaling up to reach wider populations. Gradually, the emphasis in the model on assessing impact and outcome is replaced by a focus on the processes of implementation and the extent to which successful implementation in different settings will achieve the same outcomes.

By stage 5, evaluation focuses on the scale-up (dissemination) process and on maximising the population-wide *reach* of the intervention. This requires an understanding of implementation in different contexts, and a relative decrease in focus on assessing outcomes. Stage 6, when a program is already widely adopted, is the phase of program sustainability and institutionalisation. This phase highlights the importance of continued monitoring of program delivery but distinguishes between this more routine quality-assurance process and the more formal research and evaluation methods required in the earlier stages.

Figure 2.1 Building evidence for public health programs: stages of research and evaluation

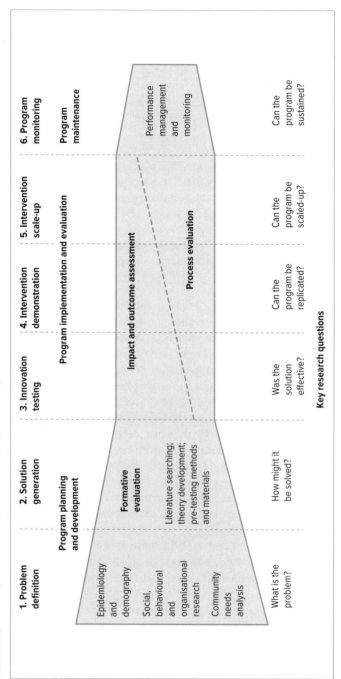

The model demonstrates that different, but connected, research methods contribute to health promotion planning and evaluation. These range from epidemiological studies (stage 1) to program planning and formative evaluation (stage 2), to formal evaluation trials (stage 3) and studies of the process of replication and scale-up (stages 4 to 6). Through this staged process, interventions can be optimally developed and systematically tested and, if found to be effective, widely disseminated to maximise their public health benefit. Although this sequence is considered optimal for evaluating a public health program, not all programs go through this linear pathway of evidence-generation in the real world (Indig et al. 2018).

Examples of each stage are illustrated in Table 2.2 and later chapters in the book.

Problem definition (stage 1)

This stage uses descriptive data and epidemiological evidence in program planning. In particular, it requires familiarity with routine population data (such as information on population prevalence of identifiable health risks; the use of mortality, morbidity and health services utilisation data; and the concepts of relative and *attributable population risk*). Two specialised subdisciplines, *behavioural epidemiology* (the use of epidemiological methods to understand the origins and determinants of health-related behaviours) and *social epidemiology* (which explores epidemiological evidence for socioeconomic and structural causes for preventable ill health) may define the importance (size and severity) of a health issue and investigate the potential contributory causes (correlates and determinants) of the problem.

It may also be useful to conduct needs assessments to: identify community and stakeholder concerns and priorities; identify access points to reach key individuals and populations; and enable more direct community participation in the *co-creation* of solutions. In combination, information gathered during this stage identifies the major health problems experienced within a defined population, the known causes of these problems and the scope for change in those causal and contributory factors.

The first case study for stage 1 in Table 2.2 on page 29 shows an international study of physical inactivity across European countries that identified less-active countries and some of the correlates of low physical activity (and related time spent sitting). This information is of relevance to national-level planners and policymakers. The second case study is from the Global Burden of Disease, a World Health Organization–informed process that assesses how much each behavioural, environmental or socioeconomic factor contributes to a range or chronic diseases and injury. This information is reported by region and country and can identify important local priorities for prevention.

At this stage, policy decisions focus on the priority areas for prevention within which proposed interventions can be developed and tested. Will projects be self-contained; will they focus on a specific risk or health determinant or on a small target group or community; or will they take a whole-population approach? In addition, are single projects anticipated or is a comprehensive program of activities proposed that may bring about change in the multiple determinants of the health problem?

Solution generation (stage 2)

This stage draws on reviewing the existing social and behavioural research to improve understanding of target populations and the range of personal, social, environmental and organisational characteristics that may be modifiable to form the basis for intervention. The next task is developing and testing an intervention (see Table 2.2). This stage involves evaluation tasks such as qualitative research methods engaging with stakeholders or the target population and/or *pilot testing* of intervention components. These methods of *formative evaluation* are described in Chapter 3, and comprise planning, developing and testing proposed program components. The result is to define a sequence of activities through a *logic model* or *intervention map* (IM) (see Chapter 1). Evaluation becomes more feasible once such a structured description of a project or program and its anticipated outcomes is in place.

In addition, a theory of change may be developed to understand the anticipated changes in individuals, social groups, organisations and the political process. More information on intervention theory can be found in the companion volume *Theory in a Nutshell: A Practical Guide to Health Promotion Theories* (Nutbeam et al. 2022).

For example, the first case study in stage 2 of Table 2.2 shows a study that uses theory to develop an infant feeding behaviour change program in Nepal (Locks et al. 2015). Single and focused behaviours, such as targeted infant feeding programs, may be usefully tested using theory. The second case study illustrates co-creation, the task of engaging and planning an intervention with members of the target audience and relevant stakeholders (Dyke et al. 2021).

Innovation testing (stage 3)

Ideally, evaluation of a new project or program will go through different stages to establish evidence of its success. Two different, but related, evaluation tasks can be identified: *process evaluation* (assessing the implementation of the intervention) and *impact or outcome evaluation* (assessing the effects of implementation relative to predicted impact and outcomes). These are discussed further in Chapters 3, 4 and 5. The relative importance of the two evaluation tasks will vary as an intervention goes through different stages of development. Figure 2.1 indicates the logical stages of evaluation beginning with a focused evaluation study to address the question of whether or not an intervention has achieved its desired outcomes: did it work? Studies to assess intervention effects are described as *efficacy studies* if carried out in optimal conditions and an *effectiveness study* if carried out in real-world conditions.

Studies of efficacy and effectiveness need to meet well-defined methodological standards (see Chapter 5). This type of study fits well with the scientific (research) perspective described in Table 2.1. To meet these methodological standards, studies that examine the effects of an intervention under optimal conditions are usually quite narrow in focus, and are often evaluated using substantial resources and optimal methods. This may be applicable to the type of projects described in single interventions, as shown in the case studies for stage 1 on page 29, and much harder to undertake for more complex or comprehensive programs exemplified by the case studies for stage 2. Because of the strong focus on evaluation design, efficacy studies often do not provide the quality of information about the implementation process that practitioners require to enable them to reproduce the intervention under less than optimal conditions. Hence, there is a need for further evaluation even if an intervention is shown to be successful in the best possible conditions.

The case study for stage 3 in Table 2.2 summarises an example of evidence-generating research. This experimental designed study tested the efficacy of a single intervention, delivering tailored text messages to people with diabetes, and showed positive effects on behaviours and clinical measures of improved diabetes control.

Intervention demonstration (replication) (stage 4)

The fourth stage occurs after the evidence of effectiveness has been demonstrated. In this stage, there is a shift in the evaluation methods to identify the conditions for success. Here the task is to replicate a project in circumstances that are closer to real life and that examine practice-relevant issues, such as the practicality of implementation and the extent to which a program can be adapted to meet variations in local contexts.

Replication studies are relevant to policymakers and funders because they indicate whether outcomes are achievable in circumstances closer to real life. Specifically, they consider contextual variables in health promotion practice relevant to implementation and program success. This type of study has a more balanced emphasis on both process and outcome. For example, it may indicate the importance of building community engagement, as well as clarifying what resources are required for success. This stage in the evolution of a program offers the opportunity for assessment of costs and benefits more related to real-life conditions—a real test of its *effectiveness*.

Chapter 5 describes tensions between maintaining rigour in study design to assess outcomes while ensuring that the intervention is responsive to differences in local circumstances and changes in the operating environment during the life of a project. Because the systems in which we operate are variable, most health promotion interventions require pragmatic adaptation to accommodate real-world constraints that are encountered during implementation.

The case study for stage 4 in Table 2.2 on page 30 provides an example of a replication study. Earlier research trials had demonstrated that curriculum-based interventions were effective in preventing smoking among adolescents. This study replicated this type of intervention under 'usual classroom' conditions (Nutbeam et al. 1993). A *cluster randomised controlled trial* was carried out to examine whether this intervention worked in real-world conditions. There was a control group and three intervention groups (family smoking prevention; curriculum intervention; both the family and curriculum interventions). At a 2-year follow-up, rates of regular smoking were similar across the four groups. The findings from this study were important; replicating previously effective programs in *real-world conditions* may not be as effective as the original trials suggested.

> *This is an important reminder that we cannot assume that a study that works well in one set of conditions can be transferred to a different environment with equal success.*

Intervention scale-up (dissemination) (stage 5)

The fifth stage indicates a further shift in emphasis, with attention given to programs reaching many more people. Such studies evaluate population-wide program delivery systems and how and whether communities maintain innovations and build capacity. In these types of studies, the primary focus is on the process of change, and research is directed towards assessing the success of scale-up strategies. This information helps to define what needs to be done to reach whole populations, by whom, to what standard and at what cost. This type of evaluation is least common in the health promotion research literature, partly as a consequence of the small number of interventions that reach this stage of research translation.

The case study for stage 5 in Table 2.2 on page 31 shows a set of studies around sun protection and skin cancer prevention, targeting outdoor pools in the United States (US). Initial efficacy trials demonstrated the program could work and subsequent process evaluation explored the scale-up of this intervention to more than 400 pools across the US (Escoffery et al. 2009, Glanz 2011). Several different types of evaluation methods and designs are needed to evaluate and understand scale-up (see Chapter 7).

Program monitoring (stage 6)

Beyond the scale-up stage, a *program of work* will become routinely *institutionalised* in the system (stage 6 in Figure 2.1). The evaluation here is directed towards sustaining program management. These tasks include population-level monitoring of key outcomes and continuing performance monitoring of program delivery. Although this stage is not considered in detail in this book, the assessment of sustained 'quality' is an important part of health promotion practice. Methodologically, many of the tasks are similar to process evaluation. As in any system, quality control of implementation needs to conform to established methods and standards of outcome. This also requires monitoring of professional practice, combined with systems for routine surveillance of health outcomes, risk factors and key determinants for health. These may be monitored in population monitoring systems, independent of any specific project, but provide trends in indicators to demonstrate sustained activity or population-wide success or reach of such programs.

Table 2.2 Case studies of research illustrating the stages in the model using different health promotion interventions (illustrating the stages in Figure 2.1)

Stage of the model	Evaluation type	Principles underpinning case study	Case studies
Stage 1: problem definition	Formative studies to inform priority setting, and describe the magnitude of a problem and its distribution across populations	International studies of the prevalence and correlates of a chronic disease risk factor show the magnitude of the problem and differences among countries. Global Burden of Disease studies assess how much of the risk of a chronic disease is attributable to a wide range of behavioural, lifestyle and risk factors and socioeconomic conditions	Jelsma et al. (2019) described a multi-country study using representative population data to identify the proportion of adults that met the recommended physical activity and sitting time guidelines across countries. The data identify socioeconomic and demographic correlates and time trends in activity and sitting time. The Global Burden of Disease has published many studies (Murray et al. 2020), with the paper illustrating the *attributable risk* for many different components of diet as well as a large range of 87 other behavioural and environmental risks for chronic disease.

(Continued)

Table 2.2 *Continued*

Stage of the model	Evaluation type	Principles underpinning case study	Case studies
Stage 2: solution generation	Formative evaluation and research to underpin chosen intervention approaches (principles illustrated here; more detailed formative evaluation examples are in Chapter 3)	Principles of planning and using diverse information to inform health promotion (for further information see Green et al. 2022)	Locks et al. (2015) outlines a good example of mixed methods used for overall formative evaluation to develop an infant feeding program in Nepal, with the results being used in developing a behaviour change approach. Dyke et al. (2021) shows an example of general principles of formative evaluation. This study describes working with adolescent girls in Tanzania, Madagascar and the Philippines to co-create a nutrition program, demonstrating timing, structural issues and solutions.
Stage 3: innovation testing	Impact/outcome evaluation (*efficacy testing* in a small sample using controlled conditions)	Testing tailored text messaging for 366 people with diabetes (randomised controlled trial)	The intervention by Dobson et al. (2018) showed improved health behaviours, perceptions of diabetes support and health outcomes (improved HBA1C measure, indicating better diabetes control).
Stage 4: intervention demonstration	Impact/process (assessing implementation and effects when delivered in diverse settings)	Replication of previously demonstrated effective smoking-prevention interventions 'in real-world conditions with usual classroom teachers'	Previous efficacy research had shown curriculum-based interventions reduced youth smoking. The Nutbeam et al. (1993) cluster trial randomised schools to controls or to three intervention arms. Rates of smoking adoption were similar across all four groups.

Stage of the model	Evaluation type	Principles underpinning case study	Case studies
Stage 5: intervention scale-up (dissemination)	Process evaluation of health promotion programs to reach more people (following efficacy/ effectiveness demonstration)	This older set of series (in the 2000s) of 'Pool Cool' interventions in the US targeted sun protection practices at swimming pools; they started with efficacy trials and moved to scaled-up (dissemination) studies	Escoffery et al. (2009) described scale-up (dissemination) of Pool Cool sun protection programs to more than 400 pools across the US. Evaluation methods included implementation surveys, environmental audits and key informant surveys (to understand barriers and facilitators to scale-up). This is also described in Glanz's 2011 summary paper.
Stage 6: program monitoring	Quality control monitoring and institutionalisation	Accepted prevention or health promotion intervention becoming routine in practice and implemented across the population	Examples in many countries include routine childhood immunisation, banning smoking or alcohol advertising and providing low-cost screening programs for at-risk age groups or populations (secondary prevention).

2.4 Quantitative and qualitative methods in program evaluation

Almost all the research discussed in this chapter can be categorised as using quantitative or qualitative methods. *Quantitative* methods are based on statistical principles and require the quantifiable measurement of phenomena. This is useful for determining the efficacy or effectiveness of a project or program. The challenge of developing reliable and valid measurements in health promotion is addressed in Chapter 5. By contrast, *qualitative* research involves methods for examining, analysing and interpreting observations to discover underlying meanings of, and patterns in, relationships. It is especially useful for explaining implementation and/or observed program effects. Both quantitative and qualitative methods can contribute to each of the research stages described. In many circumstances, they are synergistic and good-quality evaluation has components of both (Bartholomew et al. 2016).

Quantitative and qualitative methods in health promotion

Quantitative methods underpin much evidence-generating research in health promotion. These methods focus on numeric data and allow a researcher to test hypotheses comparing some attribute between groups, the assessment of changes over time or the association between two or more measures. In this approach, statistical testing (based on the probability of finding a statistically significant difference) informs the researcher. A statement that the improvement over time is 'significant' means that it is unlikely to be due to chance or random variation alone. The differences between intervention and control groups can be assessed for statistical significance, and an estimate can be made of the intervention *effect size*. Quantitative research follows a set of logical steps, from describing a testable research hypothesis, through the steps of research design, data collection, data analysis and interpretation, to finally reaching a conclusion.

On the other hand, qualitative research methods have their historical roots in social sciences such as anthropology and political science. Methods include the use of focus groups (*structured discussions* with stakeholders or members of a target group) or directly learning from participating in or with target group members (ethnographic research or participant observation, sometimes called '*action research*'). The processes of good qualitative research are the same as for quantitative research, moving through logical steps from identifying a clear research question to data collection, data analysis and interpretation. The data (information generated from this process) need to be analysed to give them structure but are not directly amenable to statistical analysis. Thus, the original hypothesis (the idea that something may change following a health promotion intervention) is not proven or refuted through statistical analysis alone, but rather through the interpretation of the researcher, based on the rules for good conduct of qualitative research.

Qualitative methods are useful where information needs to be elicited from individuals or groups that is not already well known. For example, people in project 2 on page 17 may have culturally specific beliefs about screening that will affect the likelihood of their participating in any program. Qualitative methods are efficient at eliciting these beliefs or concerns, and this understanding could improve program delivery and the development of more relevant measures to assess program effects. Qualitative research methods may also be useful to understand community members' perceptions of the effectiveness of a program or understand their views of barriers or facilitators to participation.

In some circumstances, statistical data are not required. For example, in project 3 on page 17 a community-wide healthy nutrition program was proposed; here, stakeholder interviews with local restaurant owners could inform the implementation of healthy menu choices in their restaurants. Where both qualitative and quantitative data are collected, the quantitative data can corroborate the qualitative findings, or vice versa. This so-called *triangulation* of information from different sources can be a powerful tool in understanding health promotion program effects.

Qualitative methods use data collection techniques that allow a diversity of responses, which provides a broad range of both expected and unexpected information for program planning and assessment. Additional qualitative process evaluation information collected following a program contributes to a better understanding of why the program worked and to define which program elements were perceived as successful.

Despite this, qualitative research is frequently underused. This is partly due to a values system that gives quantitative research higher status and tends to devalue qualitative research, frequently referred to as 'soft' research. As a consequence such methods may be either inappropriately applied or, when properly applied, inappropriately assessed.

As indicated above, qualitative research can be planned and rigorously executed. Identification of aims, selection and sampling of subjects, method of investigation and analysis of results can be as well defined and described in qualitative research. This overview reveals that the best approach often uses both qualitative and quantitative methods. Neither are 'soft' methods.

> *Since health promotion programs can involve complex, multi-component interventions at many levels, it is often appropriate to consider the effects of the program using both quantitative and qualitative perspectives.*

2.5 Summary

Formative, process and impact evaluation form the central focus of the following chapters, building on Chapter 1, which introduced the idea of a continuous process of evaluation from initial program conceptualisation and continues until after the program has finished. Evaluation continues beyond initial evidence-generating studies, to assess the intervention as it is replicated in other settings and scaled-up to reach more people.

The level of evaluation depends on the purposes of the intervention and also on its innovation. New programs that have never been tested should be assessed for their effectiveness; existing programs that have been trialled elsewhere should be monitored to demonstrate that they are delivering programs of a consistent quality. Health promotion interventions set up as research studies, and large-scale, expensive program interventions warrant greater investment in impact or outcome evaluation, which may require substantial research and financial support.

Evaluation of health promotion interventions is a complex enterprise and is often done poorly, using evaluation methods and measures inappropriate for the stage of an intervention's development. Many of the problems practitioners face in evaluating health promotion activity stem from unreasonable expectations of both the activity and the evaluation. Not all programs need to be evaluated to the same level of intensity or using the same evaluation designs. The stages of evaluation shown in Figure 2.1 indicate how the evaluation question, designs and methods change as a program evolves. The relative importance of formative, process and impact or outcome evaluations will vary as the research question and purpose of evaluation change.

Both qualitative and quantitative research methods contribute to successful evaluations. The use of a range of data and information sources generally provide more illuminating and relevant evidence of effects than a single 'definitive' study. Evaluations must be tailored to suit the activity and circumstances of individual programs: no single method can be 'right' for all programs.

References

Bartholomew Eldredge LK, Markham CM, Ruiter, RAC, et al. (2016). Planning Health Promotion Programs: An Intervention Mapping Approach, 4th edn. Wiley, Hoboken, NJ.

Dobson R, Whittaker R, Jiang Y, et al. (2018). Effectiveness of text message based, diabetes self-management support programme (SMS4BG): two arm, parallel randomised controlled trial. BMJ May 17;361:k1959.

Dyke E, Pénicaud S, Hatchard J, et al. (2021). Girl-powered nutrition program: key themes from a formative evaluation of a nutrition program co-designed and implemented by adolescent girls in low- and middle-income countries. Current Developments in Nutrition 5(7):1–13.

Escoffery C, Glanz K, Hall D, et al. (2009). A multi-method process evaluation for a skin cancer prevention diffusion trial. Evaluation and the Health Professions 32(2):184–203.

Glanz K (2011). Scale-up research: challenges and lessons learned from the Pool Cool diffusion trial. Annals of Behavioral Medicine 41:S153-S.

Green LW, Gielen AC, Ottoson JM, et al. (2022). Health program planning, implementation, and evaluation: creating behavioral, environmental, and policy change. Johns Hopkins University Press.

Indig D, Lee K, Grunseit A, et al. (2018). Pathways for scaling up public health interventions. BMC Public Health Dec;18(1):1-68.

Jelsma JG, Gale J, Loyen A, et al. (2019). Time trends between 2002 and 2017 in correlates of self-reported sitting time in European adults. PLoS One 14(11):e0225228.

Locks LM, Pandey PR, Osei AK, et al. (2015). Using formative research to design a context-specific behaviour change strategy to improve infant and young child feeding practices and nutrition in Nepal. Maternal & Child Nutrition 11(4):882-96.

Murray CJ, Aravkin AY, Zheng P, et al. (2020). Global burden of 87 risk factors in 204 countries and territories, 1990-2019: a systematic analysis for the Global Burden of Disease Study 2019. The Lancet 396(10258):1223-49.

Nutbeam D, Harris E & Wise M (2022). Theory in a Nutshell: A Practical Guide to Health Promotion Theories, 4th edn. McGraw-Hill, Sydney.

Nutbeam D, Macaskill P, Smith C, et al. (1993). Evaluation of two school smoking education programmes under normal classroom conditions. BMJ 306:102-7.

3

Formative evaluation

Formative evaluation comprises the set of evaluation steps before launch or implementation of an intervention. Formative evaluation includes defining the need for the intervention, developing a 'best practice' intervention using available information, consulting with the target population and bringing these stages together into a program plan.

3.1 Formative evaluation: testing methods and materials before starting a project or program of work

Chapters 1 and 2 have shown that the evaluation cycle for a health promotion program starts with the generation of ideas to solve identified public health problems. These ideas may emerge from analysis of the epidemiological information, from previously published scientific literature, from colleagues' experiences or from other sources. The initial intervention concept needs to be tested and developed. This first stage of evaluation is described as *formative evaluation*, which is the set of activities designed to define the key elements of an intervention and pre-test intervention materials and methods. This is distinct from *process evaluation*, which is a subsequent set of activities to assess program implementation (described in Chapter 4).

Formative evaluation occurs as part of program planning and takes place before the intervention is launched; everything that occurs before the start (to the left of the launch in Figure 3.1) is 'formative'. This comprises the stages from initial concept, through development, testing and refinement to the final planned intervention.

In considering program planning in Chapter 1, we recognised that practitioners often find themselves under pressure to deliver an intervention quickly and may neglect the preparatory work required before a project starts. However, formative evaluation is an essential part of good practice in program development.

Formative evaluation normally occurs in consultation with stakeholders and/or with members of the target community. Formative evaluation uses a diverse range of quantitative and qualitative methods to define and test the elements likely to be effective in an intervention.

Figure 3.1 Stages showing formative, process and impact/outcome evaluations

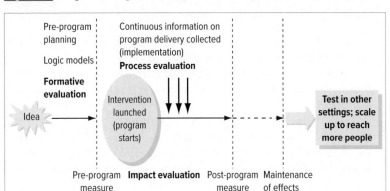

Several types of activities fall into the category of formative evaluation. These include the following.

1. Reviewing the problem and assessing previous efforts to address it. This is the initial step in formative evaluation and consists of identifying that the problem is of sufficient magnitude and importance in the target population or community to warrant public health intervention. All sources of community and population data can be used here. In addition, non-health data, such as information about the physical environment, existing facilities, socioeconomic deprivation, and local cultural and linguistic groups can all contribute to planning an intervention.

    The next step is reviewing the literature to identify effective 'good practice' examples of similar interventions in the literature or to identify research summarising effects across studies (see Box 3.1 and also Chapter 9 for further mention of evidence summaries and 'systematic reviews').

BOX 3.1: The role of reviews in identifying 'best practice'

One of the stages in formative evaluation is identifying the evidence underpinning the proposed program. Central to this is the identification of similar interventions shown to be effective. If there are many studies, it is important to ascertain if there are summaries of interventions in this area that might provide information on 'best practice'. This is derived from both formal scientific evidence reviews and practice-based reports (Green et al. 2022), but the former is typically the starting point in program planning. Reviews are particularly useful to policymakers and

(Continued)

BOX 3.1: *Continued*

practitioners as they provide summary evidence that might have application across a range of settings and populations.

There are several types of reviews. *Narrative reviews* describe 'what is in the literature' and may be time bound ('rapid reviews') or a broader overview of what is in the literature ('scoping reviews'). *Realist reviews* are interpretative and attempt to explore the mechanisms that explain how a program works (Nielsen et al. 2021). *Systematic reviews* need to be clearly identified through online databases and search strategies and are a more formal scientific and replicable process. They compare the evidence across interventions addressing the same issue and use standard methods to compare studies. They sometimes can be used to produce formal estimates of program effects using statistical techniques of meta-analysis.

A summary of evidence from available reviews can help to identify if there are sufficient papers to make a more confident judgment on the likely success of an intervention in specified circumstances, and to identify interventions and their components that are most effective in achieving outcomes.

These more formal systematic reviews, where available, can be used in program planning and formative evaluation in a number of ways.

- Provide evidence across observational studies to inform program development. For example, evidence that sugar-sweetened beverages (SSBs) lead to weight gain in children and adults (Luger et al. 2018) would indicate the need for interventions to target SSB reduction.
- Indicate that the actual evidence base may be inconclusive. For example, the apparent association between individual or community social capital and health outcomes is a widely held view, but insufficient good evidence exists, despite decades of health promotion research (Nakhimovsky et al. 2016).
- Identify interventions that may widen inequalities. For example, Lorenc and colleagues (2013) reported that some interventions (e.g. some mass media campaigns and workplace smoking bans) may widen inequalities in the outcomes, whereas other interventions narrow health inequalities.
- Identify effective attributes of interventions. For example, Visscher and colleagues (2018) described the effective components of 23 health literacy interventions.

- Summarise interventions, sometimes finding strong evidence (e.g. for mHealth interventions for chronic disease management [Lee et al. 2018]) and other times providing inconclusive evidence (e.g. for school-based mental health programs [Fenwick-Smith et al 2018]).
- Identify potential evaluation methods and outcome measures that are relevant to your planned intervention.

Information on these reviews in more detail and other examples of systematic reviews are updated regularly on the companion Evaluation website: https://evaluationinanutshell.com/.

2. Understanding the target population or community.
   Both qualitative and quantitative methods are used in formative evaluation, often to enable a participatory approach to intervention planning. In this application, formative evaluation identifies community concerns about health, may explore barriers and facilitators to action and may involve co-development of possible solutions with community members. In addition, information gathered may identify subgroups that might benefit more from an intervention. The methods include consultation with key stakeholders and/or community members, often using small-group discussions, focus groups, semi-structured interviews and prioritisation techniques for choosing among alternatives.

3. Pre-testing intervention methods and materials.
   Formative evaluation also involves pilot testing of intervention methods or materials with samples of the target audience (e.g. testing social media resources or text messages). Alternative approaches can be examined to assess which messages or resources seem to be most effective and acceptable. Pilot studies can sometimes use rigorous scientific designs including controlled trials (see Chapter 5) but can also be based on less rigorous methods to gather information on optimal approaches for delivery in the final large-scale intervention.

4. Using formative evaluation for program planning.
   Program planning is required before implementing an intervention. An example of program planning, the development of a logic model, was described in Chapter 1. Other planning techniques such as intervention mapping (IM) are used to define and describe a roadmap for the proposed program evaluation and its theory of change.

   The overall purposes of formative evaluation are to prepare the ground for delivering an intervention that is the best possible, will be most acceptable to the community or target population and will be most likely to improve health and meet community needs. Formative evaluation can assess whether a program is ready for evaluation; this is known as 'evaluability assessment' (Leviton et al. 2010). The results of formative evaluation do not imply that a guaranteed effective program will follow; it is an important step in intervention development and testing. Further adaptations are often needed during the delivery of a program.

Table 3.1 on pages 41–2 provides illustrative case studies of health promotion interventions that used different types of formative evaluation to test interventions, shape intervention methods and develop materials. These case studies illustrate the range of research methods and settings for formative evaluation.

> *Undertaking formative evaluation will significantly determine the likelihood of subsequent success and failure as well as build a sound basis for the chosen process and outcome evaluation methods.*

The first set of examples show the use of formative evaluation in identifying effective interventions, building on the types of reviews described in Box 3.1. The second set of examples aim to understand the community and its needs (e.g. in planning maternity services in Zambia [Scott et al. 2018]). Formative evaluation can be used to develop and test tools and measures and to co-develop projects with members of the target community (Dyke et al. 2021). Sometimes this formative evaluation will expose differences in the interpretation of priorities for action between 'experts' compared to the perceptions or needs of the target group.

> *Understanding the needs of the target audience, and using formative research to develop appropriate and accepted intervention methods and materials, are an essential first step in designing an effective intervention. Involving stakeholders and funders at this formative stage will also make a sustainable intervention more likely.*

Researchers also use formative evaluation to test pilot interventions. In Table 3.1, published examples include a small randomised trial to pilot test a lifestyle intervention for young men (Ashton et al. 2017), assess whether training of community workers to deliver a program is feasible (Askari et al. 2018) and test out different text messages to determine which are most effective in communicating with new mothers (Prieto et al. 2017).

Finally, examples of program planning through IM and logic models are shown at the end of Table 3.1. The first example uses IM to plan a theoretically-based telehealth program for stroke survivors (Sakakibara et al. 2017). Testing theories relevant to health promotion is further described in the companion publication, *Theory in a Nutshell* (Nutbeam et al. 2022). The last example demonstrates the use of logic models and frameworks to plan a community anti-smoking program (Khan et al. 2021).

Table 3.1 Examples of the uses of formative evaluation in health promotion

Type of formative evaluation	Author (year)	Research methods used	Use of formative evaluation results
1. *Reviewing previous solutions to the problem*			
Scoping reviews	Lentferink et al. 2017	Review of eHealth interventions (self-tracking, eCoaching)	Identified effective components of eHealth interventions
	Kotlar et al. 2021	Review of the impact of COVID-19 on maternal and perinatal health	Identified effects on pregnancy, maternal mental health, income—provides areas for project development
Systematic reviews	See Box 3.1 for examples		
2. *Understanding the target population or community*			
Formative evaluation of maternity services in Zambia	Scott et al. 2018	Needs assessment and consultations with women, community elders and healthcare workers	Undertook qualitative and quantitative research to understand the community and inform the development of services
Co-development of program with target	Dyke et al. 2021	Development of a nutrition education program in four low-middle-income countries	Worked with adolescents in each country to co-design and develop the nutrition program

(Continued)

Table 3.1 *Continued*

Type of formative evaluation	Author (year)	Research methods used	Use of formative evaluation results
3. Pre-testing intervention methods and materials			
Pilot randomised controlled trial (RCT) to decide on optimal materials and methods	Ashton et al. 2017	Pilot RCT with 50 young men of a lifestyle and mental health intervention	Results assessed feasibility, usage and engagement, and preliminary effect sizes
Community-based participatory research (CBPR)—training of community workers	Askari et al. 2018	Training of local promoters in dementia awareness	Evaluated capacity building among promoters (pilot quantitative impact data and also qualitative focus groups)
Text messages to mothers about newborn care	Prieto et al. 2017	Testing text messages and other intervention components to mothers	Evaluated by focus groups—formative evaluation informs further program development
4. Using formative evaluation for program planning			
Intervention mapping (IM) of a chronic disease management program	Sakakibara et al. 2017	Patient-centred telehealth program for stroke survivors informed by IM methods	Based on social cognitive and control theories, steps in IM guided program development and plan for implementation
Logic model framework for anti-smoking program	Khan et al. 2021	Logic model for regional Australian comprehensive smoking cessation program	Framework, especially informed development of process evaluation

'Formative research' in the literature and 'process evaluation' in this book

Some researchers use the term 'formative evaluation' to describe 'program improvement', as well as program development. In this book, assessing 'program improvement during delivery' is considered part of 'process evaluation', as it occurs after the start or launch of the intervention (Figure 3.1). Sometimes, the term formative evaluation is used to encompass both the pre-program development of an intervention and its subsequent implementation, as illustrated in a communicable disease prevention program in South Africa (Odendaal et al. 2016). In this book we confine formative evaluation to pre-intervention activity. Understanding the implementation of an intervention is a part of process evaluation (Chapter 4). Use of Figure 3.1 can resolve the issue of whether a set of evaluation tasks should be described as 'formative' or 'process', based on when the evaluation information was collected.

3.2 Formative evaluation for different types of health promotion intervention

Formative evaluation applies to many contexts and types of intervention. Behavioural researchers use formative evaluation to validate behavioural measures of intermediate variables and program outcomes, test interventions in pilot studies and assess program feasibility (Baranowski et al. 2009).

Mass media campaigns use formative evaluation to develop and test messages prior to delivery of the mass-reach communication. Social media, text messages and other digital media can also be pre-tested in formative studies. Environmental and policy interventions use formative research to develop measures that might indicate success in influencing the physical or social environment, measuring community partnership and social capital, and testing the community acceptability of innovative infrastructure changes.

Formative evaluation is also useful in large-scale, multi-component health promotion programs. Here, formative evaluation might include stakeholder consultations to identify context differences for implementation. Even when programs are scaled up to reach larger populations, formative evaluation can assess the conditions for increasing the reach of the intervention, through formative research with stakeholders and policymakers. This indicates that formative evaluation can and should occur prior to implementing an efficacy study (stage 3 in Figure 2.1) or prior to a replication or scale-up study (stages 4 and 5 in Figure 2.1). A useful model for formative research prior to dissemination and scale-up can be found in O'Hara and colleagues (2014).

3.3 Summary

Practitioners are often under pressure to deliver a program quickly with insufficient time to conduct preparatory (formative) work before the start of a program. In order to implement best practice programs, formative evaluation is an important first step in the planning and evaluation process. Undertaking formative evaluation will affect the likelihood of subsequent success or failure, as well as building a sound basis for subsequent process and outcome evaluation.

Using qualitative and quantitative research methods, formative evaluation tests program components and determines the program's relevance for the target population. Formative evaluation provides program planners with information regarding the feasibility of a program, and logic models provide a roadmap for implementation. In practical terms, formative evaluation enables the development of the best possible intervention and provides valuable information on choosing evaluation methods and outcome measurements.

References

Ashton LM, Morgan PJ, Hutchesson MJ, et al. (2017). Feasibility and preliminary efficacy of the 'HEYMAN' healthy lifestyle program for young men: a pilot randomised controlled trial. Nutrition Journal Dec;16(1):1–7.

Askari N, Bilbrey AC, Garcia Ruiz I, et al. (2018). Dementia awareness campaign in the Latino community: a novel community engagement pilot training program with Promotoras. Clinical Gerontologist 41(3):200–8.

Baranowski T, Cerin E & Baranowski J (2009). Steps in the design, development and formative evaluation of obesity prevention-related behavior change trials. International Journal of Behavioral Nutrition and Physical Activity 21(6):6.

Dyke E, Pénicaud S, Hatchard, J, et al. (2021). Girl-powered nutrition program: key themes from a formative evaluation of a nutrition program co-designed and implemented by adolescent girls in low- and middle-income countries. Current Developments in Nutrition 5(7): nzab083.

Fenwick-Smith A, Dahlberg EE & Thompson SC (2018). Systematic review of resilience-enhancing, universal, primary school-based mental health promotion programs. BMC Psychology 6(1):30.

Green LW, Gielen AC, Ottoson JM, et al. (2022). Health Program Planning, Implementation, and Evaluation: Creating Behavioral, Environmental, and Policy Change. Johns Hopkins University Press.

Khan A, Green K, Khandaker G, et al. (2021). How can a coordinated regional smoking cessation initiative be developed and implemented? A programme logic model to evaluate the 10,000 Lives health promotion initiative in Central Queensland, Australia. BMJ Open 11(3).

Kotlar B, Gerson E, Petrillo S, et al. (2021). The impact of the COVID-19 pandemic on maternal and perinatal health: a scoping review. Reproductive Health 18(1).

Lee JA, Choi M, Lee SA, et al. (2018). Effective behavioral intervention strategies using mobile health applications for chronic disease management: a systematic review. BMC Medical Informatics and Decision Making 18(1):12.

Lentferink AJ, Oldenhuis HKE, De Groot M, et al. (2017). Key components in eHealth interventions combining self-tracking and persuasive eCoaching to promote a healthier lifestyle: a scoping review. Journal of Medical Internet Research 19(8).

Leviton LC, Khan LK, Rog D, et al. (2010). Evaluability assessment to improve public health policies, programs, and practices. Annual Review of Public Health 31:213–33.

Lorenc T, Petticrew M, Welch V, et al. (2013). What types of interventions generate inequalities? Evidence from systematic reviews. Journal of Epidemiology and Community Health 67(2):190–3.

Luger M, Lafontan, M, Bes-Rastrollo, M, et al. (2018). Sugar-sweetened beverages and weight gain in children and adults: a systematic review from 2013 to 2015 and a comparison with previous studies. Obesity Facts 10(6):674–93.

Nakhimovsky SS, Feigl AB, Avila C, et al. (2016). Taxes on sugar-sweetened beverages to reduce overweight and obesity in middle-income countries: a systematic review. PLoS ONE 11(9). doi:10.1371/journal.pone.0163358

Nielsen JH, Melendez-Torres GJ, Rotevatn TA, et al. (2021). How do reminder systems in follow-up screening for women with previous gestational diabetes work? A realist review. BMC Health Services Research 21(1).

Nutbeam D, Harris E & Wise M (2022). Theory in a Nutshell: A Practical Guide to Health Promotion Theories, 4th edn. McGraw-Hill, Sydney.

O'Hara BJ, Phongsavan P, King L, et al. (2014). 'Translational formative evaluation': critical in up-scaling public health programmes. Health Promotion International Mar 1;29(1):38–46.

Odendaal W, Atkins S & Lewin S (2016). Multiple and mixed methods in formative evaluation: Is more better? Reflections from a South African study. BMC Medical Research Methodology 16(1):1–12.

Prieto JT, Zuleta C & Rodríguez JT (2017). Modeling and testing maternal and newborn care mHealth interventions: a pilot impact evaluation and follow-up qualitative study in Guatemala. Journal of the American Medical Informatics Association 24(2):352–60.

Sakakibara BM, Lear SA, Barr SI, et al. (2017). Development of a chronic disease management program for stroke survivors using intervention mapping: the stroke coach. Archives of Physical Medicine and Rehabilitation 98(6):1195–202.

Scott NA, Vian T, Kaiser JL, et al. (2018). Listening to the community: using formative research to strengthen maternity waiting homes in Zambia. PLoS ONE 13(3).

Visscher BB, Steunenberg B, Heijmans M, et al. (2018). Evidence on the effectiveness of health literacy interventions in the EU: a systematic review. BMC Public Health 18(1). doi:10.1186/s12889-018-6331-7

4

Process evaluation

Process evaluation comprises the set of activities surrounding project or program implementation, acceptance and population reach. It describes how the program is carried out in practice and helps to understand why it did or did not achieve its anticipated outcomes. This chapter focuses on process evaluation within efficacy/effectiveness testing. Process evaluation in subsequent stages of replication or dissemination is further considered in Chapter 7.

4.1 Assessing the implementation of health promotion projects and programs

Process evaluation is the set of activities directed towards assessing progress in the implementation of a project or program. Process evaluation describes and explains what happens once the project or program has actually started (see Figure 3.1), and contributes to an understanding of how and why interventions work and which elements contribute to their effectiveness. Process evaluation can also help explain negligible effects (why interventions do *not* work). It is often conducted concurrently with *impact* evaluation (see Figure 3.1). Planning for process evaluation occurs before the intervention starts and needs to be well established and integrated into the evaluation frameworks developed through intervention maps (IM) or logic models (see Chapter 1).

A broad range of activities comprise process evaluation. Process evaluation identifies whether target groups were exposed to and participated in the intervention and whether stakeholders and partners engaged with it. It also encompasses assessment of the short-term *health promotion outcomes* (described in Chapter 1, Section 1.5). The achievement of these outcomes is part of the 'process' leading to longer term impact and outcomes that are described in Chapter 1.

The aims of process evaluation are to understand how the program worked, what happened in 'real life' and how people reacted to it.

Understanding the processes of how change occurs is a fundamental aspect of any health promotion program evaluation. It is unrealistic to expect a program to succeed if it has not engaged key stakeholders, involved the community or reached the target groups as intended.

Process evaluation occurs across all stages of building evidence in Figure 2.1 and throughout intervention testing to assess effectiveness or efficacy. If a program is not delivered, endorsed or engaged with by communities, it is unlikely to have a substantial impact. It is also used to understand the replication and scale-up of programs to wider settings (stages 4 and 5, shown in Figure 2.1) to identify whether the effective parts of the program (e.g. adherence to an intervention curriculum) are maintained when the program has been disseminated in multiple field settings (see Chapter 7).

Disappointingly, process evaluation is often not carried out, or is not conducted to a high standard. For understandable reasons (such as pressure to demonstrate results), evaluation resources are often channelled into impact and outcome assessment. This means that often we do not know how well a program was implemented, and consequently may not be able to explain why it was successful or unsuccessful in achieving defined outcomes. This information is especially useful for practitioners. If a program has been successful, good process evaluation will identify how and why it worked. Alternatively, if a program fails to achieve predetermined outcomes, process evaluation can help to identify the potential causes and support subsequent modification to make future success more likely.

Monitoring program implementation is important to managers. It is a quality-assurance tool, providing ongoing feedback on program implementation and identifying possible improvements in program delivery. Process evaluation can also identify whether resources were adequate for implementation, and whether the program could be repeated elsewhere or whether different investments, different population groups or alternative programs should be considered. The elements of process evaluation are built from the logic model stages of 'activities', inputs (actions) and health promotion outcomes (see Chapter 1).

Process evaluation can comprise a broad range of methods and measurements, but common elements include the following.

- Exposure: assessing how aware participants are of the issue, program and/or message.
- Participation: identifying how well individuals, groups and organisations were recruited to and engaged in the program. This could include recruitment of end-users with a defined health problem, community members or recruitment at the organisational level such as schools, worksites or partner non-government organisations (NGOs). Low participation may lead to poorer results or to selection effects that influence interpretation of program effects (see Chapter 5).

- Engagement of the delivery system and delivery agents: assessing whether the program was delivered across the community using the predetermined methods and materials (known as *program fidelity*).
- Program satisfaction and usage: considering the extent to which participants used the resources or participated in activities as intended, and whether participants found these program elements to be relevant and useful to their needs (note that use of the program is much more important than 'program satisfaction', which is subject to social desirability bias, especially if asked immediately after a program by those who delivered the program).
- Context: examining whether the program was implemented differently in different environments, and to understand why differences occurred in different settings. This comprises an examination of the contexts in which the program was delivered, considering social influences, community opinion, economic factors, climate and changes in the physical environment, all of which may have an impact on participation and delivery.
- Variations: assessing how changes from the original protocol and adaptation of the intervention to local conditions, which are common in health promotion programs, may influence their eventual effectiveness. Standardised recording of methods and materials in delivering an intervention may help to explain subsequent outcomes.

4.2 Methods for conducting process evaluation

Table 4.1 provides some practical steps in conducting real-world process evaluation. These are process evaluation components that practitioners might consider in any health promotion program. Most of these activities involve collecting information: keeping records of program activity, conducting audits of program attendance and participation, and keeping structured records of stakeholder engagement. There are no fixed rules on which intervention elements to monitor, but all clearly articulated components of the program's logic model or intervention map should be monitored.

Researchers often quantify the amount of the program that was delivered as intended (program *exposure and dose*), the reach of the program (*proportion of the eligible target group that participates*) and the extent to which the program was delivered as intended (the *fidelity* of program delivery). For example, if half the target group only attended two out of four sessions and one-fifth attended none, then 'dose of intervention received' can be accurately described, and outcomes examined in relation to program exposure.

The reach of the program is important for understanding 'generalisability', a measure of how well the program participants represent the general population. Low reach may suggest that selected volunteers attended programs and that observed effects may be limited to motivated subgroups. Those less likely to attend or participate are often disadvantaged or marginalised subgroups, and it is important to quantify their participation because additional services or different programs may be required to meet their needs.

Table 4.1 Practical tasks in carrying out process evaluation tasks

Process evaluation tasks	Examples of what practitioners could actually do
Exposure to the intervention/ elements of the intervention	■ Assess 'exposure' by quantitative surveys or by qualitative focused discussions or interviews with target group members or stakeholders to identify their awareness of and engagement with the program.
Participation: including measures of 'recruitment' to the program, 'reach into a population', engagement and program satisfaction	■ Identify in advance how many people are expected to participate, count numbers actually attending or participating, and assess 'representativeness' (i.e. are participants similar to the whole at-risk population).
	■ Keep a record of numbers who attended all sessions or events. Document specific subgroups who did not attend (e.g. people without cars, people from specific cultural or language groups, frail elderly adults with reduced mobility).
	■ Measure program satisfaction and, even more importantly, engagement with and use of the intervention materials by program participants, and/or assess perceptions about the program among stakeholders.
	■ Monitor and document staff time and engagement (e.g. did it take longer to run the program in different contexts?).
Delivery of the intervention	■ Record sessions delivered and completeness of program delivery, such as qualitative records of program delivery at different sites and program 'fidelity' (was the intervention delivered as intended or how was it adapted ?).
Context of the intervention: describing the different settings and contexts in which programs are delivered	■ Keep a log of problems in program delivery reported by staff.
	■ Interview a sample of staff, stakeholders and participants about the environmental and social reasons, costs or other factors that influenced intervention implementation and delivery.
	■ Record ways in which program delivery differed across settings.

Sometimes satisfaction surveys are used as part of process evaluation, but these often suffer from social desirability bias, with many people keen to please the program staff. Such surveys will usually produce 'positive results', with participants reporting that they 'liked the program' and appreciated the efforts of those who delivered it. Unless results are interpreted carefully, satisfaction surveys will not provide quality information on the process of implementation.

Qualitative methods are often useful to identify the strengths and weaknesses of projects. Semi-structured interviews or focus groups with participants and non-participants can identify reasons for engagement, perceptions of the intervention format, or problems with access, language or program complexity that were not previously recognised. This can inform practitioners of issues *during the project,* enabling them to take corrective action.

Table 4.2 shows examples of different types of published process evaluation studies. This not a comprehensive list, but illustrates some common principles, with additional examples on the companion Evaluation website: https://evaluationinanutshell.com/. These studies show process evaluation in community health promotion and in clinical prevention programs, and illustrate the process evaluation components reported in each study. Most report mixed methods, indicating the use of both quantitative and qualitative methods in different parts of the process evaluation. Some focus on one dimension such as program fidelity in clinical settings (Bragstad et al. 2019) or factors associated with program engagement (Gebremariam et al. 2019). Several illustrate multi-level process evaluation measures, assessing the organisation, the program delivery professionals and the end-users of the program (Dobbie et al. 2019, Lachman et al. 2018, Morello et al. 2017).

Other types of process evaluation include the development of indicators and measures (Damschroder et al. 2016) or compare process indicators across projects (Limbani et al. 2019). Further examples of implementation research and process evaluation beyond the initial evidence-generating studies are discussed in Chapter 7.

Table 4.2 Examples of published process evaluation studies

Process evaluation studies	Partridge et al. 2016	Bragstad et al. 2019	Morello et al. 2017	Kelly et al. 2019	Lachman et al. 2018	Dobbie et al. 2019	Gebremariam et al. 2019
Program setting or purpose	Text messaging for weight loss	Psychosocial program post stroke	Hospital-based falls prevention	Telehealth chronic kidney disease	Reduce child maltreatment	Implement smoking prevention in schools	School-based obesity prevention
Recruitment/reach participation	+			+	+	+	
Qualitative (QL), quantitative (QT) or mixed methods	QT	Mixed	Mixed	Mixed	Mixed	Mixed	QT
Delivery/dose / usage/ acceptability	+		+	+	+	+	+
Context/fidelity / adherence		+	+	+	+	+	+
Barriers/facilitators / influences	+	+			+		+

+ indicates the presence of this process evaluation method

BOX 4.1: More complex methods to assess how interventions work

Process evaluation methods can be used by quantitative researchers to understand how programs work; this is through testing theory or theoretical mechanisms directly, using statistical methods to model program data. In particular, researchers test if there are theoretical *mediators,* through which the program exerts its effects. In addition, researchers often report *moderator* analyses, who define whether different subgroups change in different ways following an intervention (see Figure 4.1 and Bauman et al. 2002). This is illustrated in Figure 4.1, with the upper panel asking if a tobacco prevention program leads directly to a change in smoking status, or whether the intervention changes some intermediary theoretical variable (in this case, self-efficacy—i.e. self-confidence—as the 'mediator') and that increased confidence in turn leads to quitting smoking. The lower panel in the figure shows an example of *moderator analysis.* A quit-smoking program might result overall in a 20% cessation rate (intervention effects), but program effects are different in subgroups of the population. Here, quit rates are greater among women than men. In this example, gender is a moderator (what statisticians call an 'interaction', implying an interaction between gender and the program effect).

Figure 4.1 Advanced statistical modelling in process evaluation: understanding how interventions work through mediator and moderator analyses

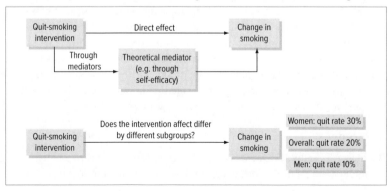

Qualitative methods are often used for understanding how programs work. These may use 'realist evaluation' techniques, that include consideration of both the context of the program and the theoretically defined mechanism which might cause end-users to change (Dalkin 2015). This approach uses a variety of qualitative methods, including in-depth discussions or interviews with end-users or stakeholders to identify the range of mechanisms through which the program may exert its effects.

4.3 Summary

Careful process evaluation provides information for understanding program implementation and mechanisms, and helps to explain program effects. Process evaluation measures what activities occur, under what conditions, by whom and with what effect. This information assists subsequent replication and scale-up studies. Information from process evaluation assists in the interpretation of impact evaluation data and the likely causal links to the program. Good process evaluation informs practitioners about successful factors in achieving defined outcomes. Through this understanding, it is possible to identify the conditions that need to be created to achieve successful outcomes.

By definition, process evaluation should occur throughout the delivery of the program. It can describe the elements in a program, assess variability in program delivery and identify the reasons for such variation. Process evaluation will also assess the reach of the program to its target audience, and the end-users' perceptions of its usefulness and relevance. Finally, process evaluation will describe the strengths and weakness of the program and explain why and how they worked or did not work.

Process evaluation should be a compulsory part of any health promotion program evaluation. Reflections on process evaluation findings can occur during an intervention, so that real-time adjustments can be made to improve the likelihood of achieving desired outcomes. In addition, process evaluation data are examined alongside outcome evaluation data at the end of the intervention to ensure the best possible understanding of what worked, with whom and under what conditions. In producing this type of information, process evaluation is also important beyond the individual project and is used in assessing implementation in scaled-up programs (see Chapter 7).

References

Bauman AE, Sallis JF, Dzewaltowski DA, et al. (2002). Toward a better understanding of the influences on physical activity: the role of determinants, correlates, causal variables, mediators, moderators and confounders. American Journal of Preventive Medicine 23(2)5–14.

Bragstad LK, Bronken BA, Sveen U (2019). Implementation fidelity in a complex intervention promoting psychosocial well-being following stroke: an explanatory sequential mixed methods study. BMC Medical Research Methodology 19(1):1–18.

Dalkin SM, Greenhalgh J, Jones D, et al. (2015). What's in a mechanism? Development of a key concept in realist evaluation. Implementation Science 10:49.

Damschroder LJ, Goodrich DE, Kim HM, et al. (2016). Development and validation of the ASPIRE-VA coaching fidelity checklist (ACFC): a tool to help ensure delivery of high-quality weight management interventions. Translational Behavioral Medicine 6(3):369–85. doi:10.1007/s13142-015-0336-x

Dobbie F, Purves R, McKell J, et al. (2019). Implementation of a peer-led school-based smoking prevention programme: a mixed methods process evaluation. BMC Public Health 19:742.

Gebremariam MK, Arah OA, Bergh IH, et al. (2019). Factors affecting the dose of intervention received and the participant satisfaction in a school-based obesity prevention intervention. Preventive Medicine Reports 15:100906.

Kelly JT, Warner MM, Conley M, et al. (2019). Feasibility and acceptability of telehealth coaching to promote healthy eating in chronic kidney disease: a mixed-methods process evaluation. BMJ Open 9(1):e024551. doi:10.1136/bmjopen-2018-024551

Lachman JM, Kelly J, Cluver L, et al. (2018). Process evaluation of a parenting program for low-income families in South Africa. Research on Social Work Practice 28(2):188–202.

Limbani F, Goudge, J, Joshi R, et al., (2019). Process evaluation in the field: global learnings from seven implementation research hypertension projects in low-and middle-income countries. BMC Public Health 19(1):1–11. doi:10.1186/s12889-019-7261-8

Morello RT, Barker AL, Ayton DR, et al. (2017). Implementation fidelity of a nurse-led falls prevention program in acute hospitals during the 6-PACK trial. BMC Health Services Research 17(1):1–10.

Partridge SR, Allman-Farinelli M, McGeechan K, et al. (2016). Process evaluation of TXT2BFiT: a multi-component mHealth randomised controlled trial to prevent weight gain in young adults. International Journal of Behavioral Nutrition and Physical Activity 13(1).

5

Evaluation methods for health promotion projects (interventions)

This chapter describes evaluation studies that generate evidence to identify if a discrete intervention works; this is stage 3 of the stages of evaluation model presented in Chapter 2. The focus of this chapter is to understand research methods used to establish if an intervention works. There is a need for balance between 'scientific' design against public health pragmatism in research design, sample selection and measurement.

Chapters 3 and 4 described the formative and process evaluation methods that support the development and implementation of a health promotion project. This chapter focuses on the evaluation designs and research methods that test the efficacy and effectiveness of a health promotion intervention. 'Efficacy' is an assessment of the outcomes of an intervention in ideal circumstances—where there was optimal delivery and a high degree of control over the intervention. 'Effectiveness' is an assessment of the success of a health promotion intervention under 'real-world' or 'field' conditions—where there is less control over the conditions that might influence success or failure.

Efficacy studies and some effectiveness studies are often smaller scale, usually conducted in selected populations of volunteers who agree to participate. These are often evaluations of discrete well-defined projects (projects usually using a single intervention strategy); for example, a social media intervention to encourage healthy eating, a school curriculum to teach young people about HIV risk, or a social cognitive theory–led behaviour change intervention to support regular smokers to quit. Chapter 6 addresses issues relating to the evaluation of more complex, multi-component health promotion programs and Chapter 7 deals with research issues around the evaluation of scaled-up studies.

5.1 Evaluation designs for health promotion projects

The term 'evaluation design' describes the set of tasks used to systematically examine the effects of a health promotion intervention. A well-conducted evaluation can provide decision-makers with confidence that the intervention caused the observed effects and that these did not occur by chance or due to other factors or influences. To achieve this, we need to ensure that:

- the program was optimally *developed and planned* (formative evaluation), *implemented* as intended, and *reached* the target audience (process evaluation)
- the processes of *recruiting people* into the intervention are described (e.g. who they were and how they were selected)
- the best possible reliable and valid *measurements* were used to assess the impact and outcomes from the intervention (the results)
- the best possible *research design* was used to assess the effects of the intervention
- no *alternative explanations* exist for the results, so that we can be confident that the results observed are attributable to the intervention
- further research may be conducted to *identify* how and why the program worked (or did not work) for the whole, or for subsets of, the target group.

The research process in an evidence-generating intervention

Figure 5.1 shows some of the key features of good evaluation methods, from initial recruitment of participants, to process and impact evaluation, to replication and dissemination (the latter are discussed in Chapter 7). The first step is to identify the group of people who enrol in the intervention.

Identification of the target group

This is the potential target group among which to seek participants for the intervention. For example, with a very large national program, the evaluation methods will be different to that testing the effects of a small, focused community project. The effects will also be influenced by the characteristics and *health literacy* of the study's self-selected participants.

It is important to identify whether participants are typical (or *representative*) of the whole population. Once the intervention begins, people are defined as 'included' in an intervention or program, and from that point onwards, process and impact evaluation are carried out. After the intervention has concluded, follow-up assessment is needed to assess short- and long-term impact and outcomes. The concept of participation is important to understanding the potential for a program's results to be *generalised* to other settings. The starting point is identifying people who are eligible for an intervention. For example, a smoking-prevention intervention might target all pregnant women who smoke, but a much smaller number of women might actually enrol in the program and of these, only half might complete the intervention as planned (see Figure 5.1).

Figure 5.1 The evaluation process

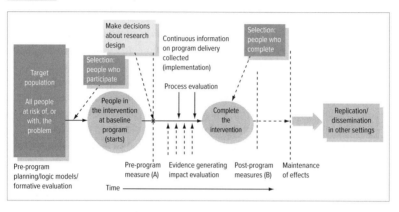

---

*It is important to assess the differences between participants who are **eligible** from those who actually **enrol** at the start of the program, and those who **complete** the program.*

Choice of evaluation (or research) designs

The next part of the research process is the choice of an evaluation design (also known as a *research design* or *study design*). Evaluation designs should provide the best possible fit with the intervention objectives and the context in which implementation takes place. For example, a program to increase the use of injury-prevention strategies in the workplace may have a different research design when compared to a community-based program to prevent falls and injuries in a group of home-bound older people.

Experimental (controlled trial) designs

There is a hierarchy of research designs from the 'most rigorous', which use *experimental* designs, most commonly *randomised controlled trials (RCTs)* and a range of quasi-experimental other methods described below. Choice of method is dictated by a range of circumstances, often related to the source and level of funding.

The RCT design is illustrated in design 1, shown in Figure 5.2. The people who receive the intervention (shown as 'X' in the figure) are not predetermined, with individuals randomly allocated to receive or not receive the program. This *random allocation* of individuals makes it more likely that differences (such as personal background or existing health status) between those receiving an intervention and those not receiving an intervention can be minimised.

Figure 5.2 Quantitative evaluation designs for individual programs (stage 3 of Figure 2.1), ranked from 'most scientific' experimental designs to less scientific 'pre-experimental' designs

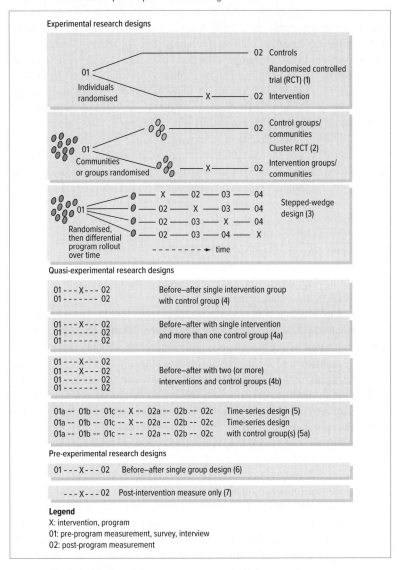

It reduces the possibility that observed changes in the intervention group are due to 'chance' effects caused by existing differences in the two populations and increases the likelihood that the intervention caused any observed changes.

Once the individuals have been randomly allocated to the *intervention or comparison (control) groups,* a baseline assessment is made of their characteristics (age, gender and the outcomes of the intervention; e.g. smoking behaviour or healthy eating patterns) to determine that the intervention and *control* groups are comparable at the beginning (baseline) assessment (shown as 'A' in Figure 5.1). Measurements are repeated on the same individuals after the intervention to assess change (shown as 'B' in Figure 5.1), and to test that change for *statistical significance.* The quality of an experimental evaluation design can be examined according to well-established criteria, such as the comprehensive 25-item CONSORT checklist (Consolidated Standards of Reporting of Trials: http://www.consort-statement.org/).

In addition to individual-level randomisation, it is possible to randomise at the level of whole communities or groups (e.g. randomising workplaces, primary care centres or schools to receive an intervention); this is known as a cluster RCT (panel 2, Figure 5.2, and Table 5.1). This may be necessary because, within the same school, students are likely to share common influences on their health behaviour or beliefs, which means we need to take account statistically of this clustering. This research design is well-suited to interventions that are intended to be delivered to whole groups (such as a school class), or interventions based on a modification to the environment that might have an impact on a whole group (e.g. the introduction of healthy food options in a worksite canteen).

A third RCT design is the stepped-wedge design, where units or groups are randomly allocated sequentially to an intervention, so that waiting-list groups can be compared as the intervention rolls out across a population (panel 3, Figure 5.2, and Table 5.1). This is useful across a large region, where for financial or other practical reasons an implementation needs to be rolled out over time.

Because randomised trials usually involve some individuals receiving an intervention and some not, it is important to make sure that nobody fails to receive the care that they need. In these circumstances 'usual care' or minimal interventions are often provided. For example, in a primary care setting, we could randomly allocate people with diabetes to receive a comprehensive education and skills development program, and others allocated to a control group consisting of their 'usual clinic care'. In such circumstances it is important to follow ethical protocols and ensure that your evaluation study has received approval from an appropriate institutional ethics review board.

It is also important to keep the people in intervention and control groups separated from each other as much as is practically possible. One evaluation challenge is to ensure that there is no *contamination* of the control group. For example, sometimes those receiving an intervention can share information or program resources with control group participants, who are not intended to receive the intervention. This increases the chances that controls may make

Table 5.1 Examples of research design (additional examples are updated on the companion Evaluation website: https://evaluationinanutshell.com/)

Randomised trial designs (experimental studies)		
Individual-level RCT	Widmer et al. (2017): adding digital interventions to cardiac rehabilitation	Individuals randomised to receive additional digital intervention components showed more weight loss than controls
Individual-level RCT	Ng et al. (2015): RCT of intervention to reduce frailty in older adults	Multi-component lifestyle intervention recipients showed reduced frailty
Cluster RCT	Victor et al. (2018): RCT of hypertension advice to African-American men	Randomised barber shops (setting) to intervention/controls where advice was delivered to clients by health professionals
Stepped-wedge	Omer et al. (2021): evaluated a universal postnatal home visiting program	Rolled out intervention sequentially across eight regions in Nigeria to improve child health
Quasi-experimental evaluation studies		
Quasi-experiment	Vissenberg et al. (2017): social network enhancing intervention to low socioeconomic status people with diabetes	Non-random allocation to receive intervention; used mixed methods; intervention improved self-management behaviours more than controls
Time series	Su & Huang (2020): promoted a national screening program for colorectal cancer early detection, introduced in some regions	Interrupted time-series evaluation, screening increased following promotion, and showed lower cancer incidence compared to earlier periods
Pre-experimental designs		
Pre–post single group	Gumz et al. (2018) public health and online intervention for eating disorders (anorexia)	59 women pre–post assessment of impact of the intervention, supported by qualitative evaluation (mixed methods)
Post only	McConnell et al. (2012) evaluated the Triple P parenting program	923 parents, post-only surveys; showed program satisfaction; no evidence can be provided on program effectiveness
Qualitative-only evaluation	Tudor-Sfetea et al. (2018): evaluation of mobile apps for smoking cessation	Used qualitative methods for 29 smokers to assess reported impact on quit attempts and explain reasons for quitting

positive changes, and such contamination makes it (statistically) more difficult to detect the effects of a program. This is particularly challenging in health promotion interventions that are designed to reach whole populations—hence the use of cluster RCTs, randomising by whole settings or geographically discrete units, as a research design alternative.

Although the use of experimental designs is always preferable for evidence generation, it is often impractical to evaluate a health promotion program using an RCT design. Controlled trial designs require substantial funding and good control over the intervention delivery. This design is required when there is a high need for 'generating evidence' of intervention efficacy; for example, when a program is being tested for the first time or is expensive (and would be costly to reproduce widely), may be controversial, or is considered risky.

Quasi-experimental and pre-experimental designs

Given the diversity of settings and complexity of interventions, alternative designs may be considered. These provide less definitive evidence of program effectiveness but may be feasible and affordable. 'Best practice' in health promotion evaluation will always require pragmatic decisions balancing the 'optimal against the possible' in evaluation design. These designs are categorised as 'quasi-experimental' and 'pre-experimental' designs.

Quasi-experimental designs usually have a *control* or *comparison* population against which intervention group effects could be compared (designs 4, 4a and 4b in Figure 5.2, and Table 5.1). Here, the group(s) receiving the intervention are not randomly assigned, and the 'causal evidence' is less strong. This is especially the case when the intervention is delivered to enthusiastic volunteers who are then compared with a less motivated 'control' population.

As is the case with RCTs, the quality of the results from quasi-experimental studies is dependent on the design and research methods used. Non-randomly allocated communities or groups can sometimes be matched, and analyses can be statistically adjusted for baseline differences between intervention and control groups.

RCTs have the same individuals assessed before and after the program. Quasi-experimental studies may also involve the same people (panel or *cohort*) followed up from pre- to post-program, but some population interventions are evaluated using different (independent) *cross-sectional* representative samples of people from the target population to assess changes over time. This design is a *repeat cross-sectional study,* and while feasible in many health promotion program evaluations, it is not as methodologically strong as a cohort study for explaining how and why observed changes occurred.

Quasi-experimental designs may provide a pragmatic approach to evaluating many health promotion interventions. This is especially the case where interventions are directed at whole populations or large regions (where allocation of individuals to intervention and control groups is impossible). Examples include a region-wide immunisation program, a national mass media campaign or large-scale preventive service offered over a large region. In these examples, careful quasi-experimental designs are feasible designs for assessing program effectiveness. Examples of interventions using a quasi-experimental design are shown in Figure 5.2 designs 4, 4a and 4b.

Another type of quasi-experimental evaluation design is a *time-series design which is characterised by* multiple pre-intervention measurements, followed by the health promotion intervention, and then multiple post-intervention measurements (Figure 5.2, types 5 and 5a). Here, trends in the measure of interest can be observed at many time points before the intervention, and effects assessed by changes in the multiple observations following the intervention. An even better design has multiple time points of data also collected in a comparison region which did not receive the intervention. An example would be trends in screening rates in a region where screening was promoted, compared to rates in a comparison region. Time-series designs are also useful in the evaluation of policy interventions, as they allow for structured observation of change following the introduction of a policy (see natural experiments in Chapter 8).

The last group of designs are described as *pre-experimental*. These provide the weakest evidence and should only be used after other possibilities have been considered. A 'before–after' one-group evaluation design (*pre–post study; type 6* in Figure 5.2) is a weak design to demonstrate that an intervention *caused* any observed changes. It is often used in pilot studies to estimate the likely effect of an intervention. However, in some circumstances, a 'before–after' single group design is the only feasible design. An example would be the evaluation of a large-scale national campaign, where it is usually not possible to have a comparison population or region. This type of study design is strengthened by having multiple baseline pre-intervention measures and multiple post-intervention measures to assess program impact.

The weakest design is the one-group 'post-program only' evaluation (design 7 in Figure 5.2), where measurements are only made following the program. This design provides no evidence of program effectiveness. 'Post-only' designs may be used for collecting process evaluation measures, as these can be collected after the program has finished but should never be considered for assessing program impact.

In addition, qualitative evaluation methods including case series designs or qualitative focus group discussions could also be classified as 'pre-experimental'. Such qualitative evaluations may generate process evaluation information and contribute substantially to understanding the program and interpreting any observed effects. Occasionally, qualitative-only methods are used in program evaluation, and can be useful, although the evidence is not 'causal' (see the last row of Table 5.1).

In summary, the first stage is deciding on the best possible evaluation design to meet circumstances for a particular program evaluation. Several important technical issues must also be addressed to improve the quality of evidence provided. These include participation rates of those eligible for the program (see Table 5.2), the measurements chosen and the analytical methods used to interpret the data. Each of these is considered in the remainder of this chapter.

5.2 Selection bias and sampling

The issues surrounding selection effects relate to the way in which people from the target population end up in the 'evaluation' study and whether they are *representative* of the target population. Methods for minimising *selection bias* are shown in Box 5.1.

Sampling and recruitment

In small-scale interventions, we include everyone who volunteers for the intervention. This is a limitation of small-scale interventions, as the results may not be applicable to the general population. If small-scale interventions are found to be effective, they need to be tested in larger and more representative samples to assess whether or not the observed effects are replicated (see Chapter 7).

When planning large community-wide programs, we cannot evaluate everyone who might benefit from an intervention, so we *sample* a subset of individuals from the population to assess the impact of the program. By using *random sampling,* the effects of the program on a *random sample* can be considered applicable (generalisable) to the whole source population. Random sampling implies that a list of the target population exists, and that people can be randomly selected for the evaluation. Examples of such population-level lists include census data, health clinic or health insurance lists, employee payroll lists, lists of populations of patients registered in primary care, school lists of enrolled pupils and so on. Random sampling is best drawn using a computer-generated list of random numbers.

BOX 5.1: Minimising selection bias

The evidence generated by a study is more persuasive if the sample studied is 'typical' of (*generalisable to*) the general population. In developing a study design, it is important to minimise selection *bias* that may affect the results. Bias is where something differs systematically from the true situation or contributes to conclusions that differ from the 'true situation'. Selection biases may include the *selection* of participants (enrolment and recruitment of participants in a study/intervention, and their retention for the duration of the study). Those who enrol in an intervention may be different to those who do not participate (known as *non-response bias*); in addition, selection effects include examining the differences between those who *drop out* or do not complete the intervention with those who complete it. Completing participants may have different social, educational or other attributes which contribute to the observed effects of the intervention.

To obtain generalisable evidence, it is important to try to obtain a *representative sample* and to maintain a *high participation* rate through the intervention. Maintaining people in evaluation studies may be facilitated by not requiring too much in terms of assessment, by active support and encouragement and sometimes by providing incentives for continued participation.

In cases where no population 'list' or record exists, it will not be possible or practical to achieve a true random sample from a population (e.g. among homeless people or other highly marginalised groups). Other examples of ways in which sampling occurs are shown in Table 5.2. These include *convenient samples* of volunteers and *snowball sampling*.

Sampling techniques are used to ensure that the population being studied is representative of the whole target population, and *statistical tests* can be used to assess the importance (referred to as *significance*) of the observed changes between the intervention and comparison samples. In general, the larger the study sample is, the greater the chance of showing a statistically significant difference between the intervention and comparison groups.

Table 5.2 Sampling methods used in the evaluation of health promotion interventions

	Recruitment of participants to a small health promotion trial *(e.g. a trial of an e-intervention to increase self-management skills in people with heart disease)*	Sampling of people to evaluate a large-scale intervention *(e.g. a community program to increase the rate of cancer screening for all women aged over 50 years)*

Optimal sampling method ↑	■ Random sampling from the population of people with heart disease
	
	■ Sampling from a defined database of people with heart disease—from hospital records or heart-support non-government organisations
	
	■ Sampling from numerous community groups and clinic settings—even if non-random, may show enough diversity to be generalisable
	
	■ 'Snowball samples', where hard-to-reach individuals can be found and sampled through social networks
	
	■ Volunteers with heart disease recruited through newspaper advertisements or local hospital clinics
		■ Evaluate effects in a random sample from the population of all women aged 50+
		
		■ Other variants:
		
		  – random sampling with increased samples (oversampling) of specific groups of interest—such as a marginalised group that is less likely to be screened
		
		  – universal sampling (if the population is small, it is possible to sample everybody)
		
		■ Non-random (convenient) sampling, for example:
		
		  – street intercept samples
		
		  – samples of middle-aged women from a particular cultural or geographic grouping
		
		  – other convenience samples from women attending a club or belonging to an organisation

↓ **Least generalisable sampling method**		

5.3 Statistical significance and data analysis

A serious examination of statistical methods is beyond the scope of this book, but an understanding of some basic statistical concepts is necessary to interpret evaluation findings. Further reading is recommended at the end of this chapter. Even if good evaluation methods are used, if the data are not analysed and interpreted appropriately, the evaluation will not establish the success or otherwise of an intervention.

Sample size calculations

Initial statistical considerations occur before the program starts. We need to know how many people we need to include in a study to be confident that the results we get are likely to be true (*sample size*). For example, an obesity prevention program might aim for intervention participants to lose an average of 3 kilograms of weight over 3 months. The 3 kilogram weight loss is estimated on the basis of effects observed in previous studies and is likely to produce health benefits. With known measures (and with an understanding of their variation) it is possible to calculate the number of people needed in a study population to detect an effect of a pre-specified size. Obviously, this sample size calculation should be done before the evaluation starts, as it will guide the numbers needed to be recruited into the program.

Statistical methods and statistical testing

Statistical methods are used to determine whether the results observed are likely to be 'real' or might have occurred by 'chance'. This is referred to as the level of *statistical significance*. Statistical significance describes the probability of the observed results (i.e. the difference in a target outcome when comparing the measure before and after an intervention, and/or between intervention and control groups) occurring by chance. Statistical significance is often described in terms of probability of the observed finding occurring by chance; these statements of probability are described as *p values,* which are often shown in published papers as $p < 0.05$ or $p < 0.01$. This simply means that there is a 1-in-20 or 1-in-100 probability of an observed outcome occurring by chance respectively. A related statistical concept is the use of *confidence intervals* around an observed outcome. In this case confidence intervals describe how likely the true results in the underlying population are to be outside the range described by the confidence limits.

Statistical tests require consideration of the type and distribution of the data collected, specifically whether data are *continuous* measures or *categorical.* A continuous measure can take many values and be described in terms of an average (mean) value and its variation (standard deviation). For example, blood pressure or weight in kilograms are continuous measurements. Some outcomes are just described as a category (e.g. 'improved/did not improve'; 'smoker/non-smoker'). Different statistical methods are required to analyse continuous data (these include *parametric tests,* such as t-tests, linear regression models and so on), compared to analytical approaches to data in categories, which require the use of chi-squared statistics, and relative risks or odds ratios. These are illustrated by examples of 'continuous data' and 'categorical data' in data from a hypothetical intervention in the companion Evaluation website: https://evaluationinanutshell.com/.

Other factors influencing interpretation of results

In analysing evaluation results, we need to consider whether the results might be due to some other factors, either in the data or external to the program. Internal factors might contribute in subtle ways—it may be that one group improves most because it is more socially connected or has greater confidence about achieving the outcomes. External factors might include unpredicted media interest in an issue during an intervention, natural disasters or major events, or even global influences. These are referred to as secular trends. For example, in some countries, tobacco use has declined and community views on restricting smoking in indoor environments have strengthened over a prolonged period. Any evaluation should consider these background changes in community attitudes and behaviours, and assess whether the program could produce effects greater than these existing *secular trends.*

Similarly, the background effects of large-scale national programs may reduce or confuse the observed effect of a local-level intervention. For example, the impact of a national media campaign to promote uptake of an effective immunisation among older people might completely mask the impact of a local project conducted to improve immunisation uptake by patients in an individual health clinic.

Finally, extraneous factors associated with the intervention and with the outcomes of interest may distort the estimates of program effectiveness. These are known as *confounding factors* and should be considered in analysis. As they are somewhat technical, they are beyond the scope of this volume (see Bauman 2002).

It is worth noting that it may not always be 'positive change' that indicates program success. For example, given the increases in obesity in many countries, a local program that demonstrated no change in obesity prevalence over 5 years at the same time as national prevalence was rising would be a relative success. In such circumstances, having a control region or prior national monitoring data is useful, and allows this intervention to be appraised as a successful innovation in preventing the expected weight gain.

5.4 Health promotion measurement

A fundamental component of evaluation is the accurate measurement of impact and outcomes. Measurement can use qualitative or quantitative methods, or both. In assessing intervention effects, we aim to detect changes in health promotion outcomes such as changes in (measures of) knowledge and community attitudes; and impact on intermediate health outcome measures, such as changes in health behaviours or environments.

There are many challenges in measurement. Many measures are based on self-reported information (collected by questionnaires completed online or on paper, or by telephone or face-to-face interview). Other measures are device-based and directly observable assessments of phenomena (e.g. body weight, blood pressure or immunisation status). Measurement may be of individual attributes (knowledge, attitudes, social norms) or may assess characteristics of organisations, environments, communities or systems.

The definition and measurement of *intermediate health outcomes,* such as health behaviours and healthy environments, and the *health promotion outcomes* that may influence them, have taxed the skills of researchers for decades. Measurement development has prioritised the assessment of individual behaviours, such as smoking or alcohol use, rather than measures of health promotion processes. The latter (e.g. measures of social mobilisation or health literacy) are less well-developed.

One important issue is the difference between *measures and indicators.* Indicators are often proxy or indirect measures that reflect a generally related area and can be used on a large scale to monitor processes or progress. An example of the difference can be seen if we think about measures of, first, adolescent health, and second, social capital. For adolescents, measures might be rates of binge drinking of alcohol, illicit drug use or individual-level mental health measures; at the community level, process indicators might include education system provision, access to youth facilities, or criminal conviction rates for drug possession. Both indicators and measures should be included in an evaluation of adolescent substance use prevention interventions. Similarly, in a study to improve social capital, we might use individual-level quantitative measures, such as sense of coherence, trust and social support. In addition, we may also use community-level indicators such as poverty, crime rates and safety. In many projects, the indicators are routinely collected and used to corroborate trends in phenomena of interest to decision-makers.

Measurement reliability and validity

We need to be sure that what we measure is reliable and valid and can be sensibly used as the basis for an evaluation. Poor measurement is one source of bias that may lead to erroneous conclusions about program effects. The concept of 'measurement bias' is discussed in Box 5.2.

BOX 5.2: Measurement error and measurement bias

Measures are not perfect: there is some error in all measurement, compared to the 'true state' that is being assessed. One kind of measurement error is 'random variation', as some attributes vary naturally when measured at different times. An example of this is blood sugar, which might be higher if measured soon after a meal.

(Continued)

BOX 5.2: *Continued*

Another problem with measurement is 'bias', which is the amount that the observed measurement differs from the 'true' measurement. Sometimes we measure the 'true value' or close to it, as our only measurement; for example, cholesterol levels or immunisation status are assessed using objective measures. In other circumstances, we can ask people to report their smoking status or weight, and we can assess how much this differs from objective measurements of these phenomena. Sometimes it is difficult to know how far measures differ from the 'truth'. For example, in subjective self-report measures of 'attitudes' or 'social capital', we may need to use special techniques adapted from the social sciences (psychometric techniques) to assess measurement reliability and validity.

Poor-quality measurements can produce either *type 1* or *type 2* errors. For example, if there is a poor-quality measurement in our evaluation (one with too much random variability or one with too much bias) then error in measurement may preclude our finding a significant difference following an intervention. An example of this could be the measurement of weight—self-report may be biased, or poor scales may show too much variation. Therefore, using good, reproducible measures that are not biased is an important step in optimising evaluation methods.

Test–re-test reliability refers to the stability of a measure, assessing the extent to which each time the measure is used it will measure the same thing. The most common method used to test reliability is the repeat administration of the measurement on the same people, using the same administration procedures, within a short period of time (1 to 2 weeks).

Testing for reliability is important even when the object of study can be observed directly (e.g. when rating the characteristics of an environment, such as a park or a school). In this case, reliability can be determined by the level of agreement between two observers or 'raters' of the same phenomenon. This is known as *inter-rater reliability*. If there is inter-rater disagreement, protocols need to be developed to standardise data collection.

Validity is the assessment of the 'truth' of a measurement. A question, scale or test is considered *valid* to the extent that it measures what it intended to measure. A reliable measurement is not necessarily a valid measurement, since you may measure the wrong thing, but do so consistently (see Figure 5.3).

Validity can be assessed objectively. For example, it is possible to objectively measure cotinine in a saliva or blood sample to detect recent tobacco use. This provides a good biochemical test of the validity of self-reported questions on smoking behaviour. Although desirable, such objective measures are not always available, practical or affordable.

Measurement of attitudes and beliefs and self-efficacy do not lend themselves to such objective verification so measurement validation techniques are needed, usually using methods developed in the social sciences. These include whether the items are considered relevant by experts (referred to as *face validity*), and cover all dimensions of interest (referred to as *content validity*). It is challenging to develop valid measures of concepts such as 'social capital' or 'capacity-building' where experts do not agree on the constituent elements of the concept. This depends on an understanding of the relationship between *concepts, variables* and *constructs*. A *concept* is a theoretical idea used to describe a phenomenon that is not directly observable. Concepts must be turned into measurable *variables*, which are validly and reliably assessed and show variation among people. Variables may be single questions or *items*, or summarised as composite *scales or scores*. How well the items or questions 'fit' into the score or scale can be assessed by estimating the *internal consistency* of the items. The process of turning items into scores uses psychometric statistical techniques, which describe the measurement properties of these underlying constructs and how well the items are related to the construct. This is called *construct validity*. Examples are further described on the companion Evaluation website: https://evaluationinanutshell.com/

The importance of measurement for practitioners is to understand the principles of good measurement to assist in the critical appraisal of evidence in the published literature. Further reading, or consultation with a statistical measurement expert, is recommended before using them in a program evaluation.

The uses of measurement in evaluation

The purpose of a health promotion intervention is to produce change in a range of determinants of health and thereby improve health. To this end, a measure should be capable of changing in response to an intervention. This is known as measurement *responsiveness* or *sensitivity to change*. Responsiveness is needed in measures of a discrete behaviour, such as breastfeeding or smoking, but is also true of more subjective program outcomes. For example, for a program trying to change measures of public opinion about restricting smoking inside buildings, the measure needs to be shown to be both reliable (stable) and yet sufficiently sensitive to change in response to an intervention targeting community values in the environments in which smoking might occur.

A hypothetical time-series design in a program evaluation is shown in Figure 5.3, with monthly measurements. The figure shows the mean outcome score for two different measures of 'self-confidence' that might have been used in an intervention to improve confidence among young people. This figure shows both measurement *reliability* and *responsiveness*. Mean scores are shown on the y-axis and time in months on the x-axis. Measure 1 (solid line) is stable (*reliable*) during serial administrations over the months May to September, with the mean scores being similar, around a value of 13–14. This shows that the measure does not change in the absence of an intervention. When the intervention occurs in October, the self-confidence score shows *responsiveness,* increasing to a value of 21 immediately after the intervention.

By contrast, Measure 2 (dotted line) has poor measurement properties for two reasons. It shows great variability pre-intervention, showing substantial fluctuation (is not *reliable*), and then fails to show any *responsiveness* to the intervention. This measure will show possible effects in the absence of an intervention due to random measurement fluctuations, and will fail to show an effect when exposed to the October intervention (both *type 1 and type 2* errors); hence, its use will lead to the wrong conclusion about the program's effects.

It is almost impossible to remove all sources of error and bias from the different measurements that are used in a health promotion evaluation.

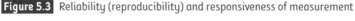 **Figure 5.3** Reliability (reproducibility) and responsiveness of measurement

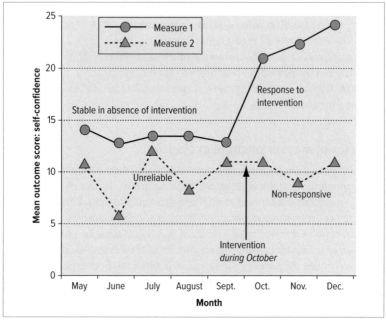

Other measurement problems and ways of addressing them are shown in Box 5.3. It is important that a researcher uses the best possible measures in evaluation and that practitioners are aware of potential measurement bias when critically assessing the quality of evidence reported in any evaluation.

BOX 5.3: Examples of other measurement issues that can influence evaluation results

- *Response bias as a consequence of simply being observed—* for example, people may report 'socially desirable' answers to sensitive issues, such as substance use, sexual behaviours or domestic violence. Even the mode of administration (e.g. comparing interview data to that collected by online anonymous questionnaires) can show different values. These biases can be reduced by using questions presented in a neutral form and by offering anonymity or confidentiality where possible.

- *Response bias as a consequence of sensitisation to the issue—*for example, where a person is asked the same questions on repeat occasions. This is particularly a risk in control populations where repeatedly asking someone about their attitudes or behaviours might influence their thinking about an issue or to take action that they might not otherwise have taken. If a person who smokes is asked in some detail about their smoking habit on repeated occasions, this might prompt him or her to attempt to quit. This bias can be reduced by undertaking independent *cross-sectional* surveys of different people before and after an intervention, rather than conducting surveys with the same *cohort*.

- *Response changes as a consequence of the maturation of a group or cohort—*for example, at the extremes of age. Longitudinal studies of adolescents may show changes in attitudes or beliefs as a consequence of growing up, which may be due to maturation processes, not an intervention. Similarly, older adults may show declines in measures of cognitive abilities or functional status as a consequence of ageing, which may attenuate any observed positive intervention effect. These changes are not necessarily a source of bias but need to be considered in the analysis of change over time in a cohort. In the same way, changes to the composition of communities over time may mean that serial cross-sectional survey samples from the same geographical area differ in sociodemographic attributes; if serial surveys are used to evaluate programs, then efforts to account for these differences are required.

Measurement across different stages of evaluation

Each stage in the planning and evaluation process may require different measures and pose different measurement challenges. In program planning, routinely collected information on mortality, morbidity and health behaviours might be used to prioritise health problems for intervention. In assessing program implementation, process evaluation measures of participation and engagement may be used. These measures might need to be specially designed for the project, or at least adapted for use from another project evaluation. Assessment of the short-term impact of a project may use established measures of knowledge, self-efficacy or social attitudes and, over time, assessing impact using the many existing measures of behaviour or the environment. Longer term health outcomes use epidemiological data on mortality and morbidity. Beyond assessment of the effectiveness of a program (stage 4 evaluation in Figure 2.1), evaluation of the quality of dissemination requires measures of spread or diffusion of the programs into communities (see Chapter 7). Examples of measures at different stages of evaluation are shown in Table 5.3.

Table 5.3 Measurement at different stages of program evaluation

Stage of program and measurement needs	Examples of measures	Measurement challenges and pitfalls
Program planning and design—formative evaluation	Measures that assess likely responses of the target group as part of program material testing; perception of stakeholders of program components	Sufficient sample variation to assess the utility of formative or pilot evaluation findings
Program implementation; process measures; implementation indicators—examples only	Measures of participant attendance, and completion; measures of program fidelity; measures of organisational partnerships or environmental changes	Reliability and validity of process measures; known measurement properties of indicators such as audits of program attendance, satisfaction measures, established measures of community partnership and engagement
Health promotion outcomes: **individual level**	Awareness of health issues; cognitive changes such as self-efficacy, intention to be more active, beliefs	Psychometric properties, test re-test repeatability and construct validation of cognitive measures, social support and social capital measures

Stage of program and measurement needs	Examples of measures	Measurement challenges and pitfalls
Supra-individual measures	Social supports; enhanced social influences; social environment; social capital (collective efficacy); organisational measures	Reliable and valid measures and indicators needed at the family, community or organisational level
Intermediate health outcomes (impact)	Behavioural changes; whether there are specific domains with each behaviour (such as different dietary components or different levels of physical activity)	Measurement properties including criterion validity (e.g. self-report diet or physical activity); whether measurement domains are part of the same construct; assessment and testing of *mediator* (and *moderator*) variables
Physical environmental measures	Changes made to physical environments completed	Validity of environmental assessments; inter-rater agreement using audit tools
Community-level change/ policy measures	Policies developed; program elements institutionalised in the (health or other) system; program elements self-sustaining	Reliability of policy measures and their implementation; replication of process and impact effects
Long-term health outcomes	Reduced morbidity or reduced disease incidence; improved wellbeing or quality of life	Validity of health outcomes or quality-of-life measures; predictive validity of intervention exposure on outcomes
Diffusion and dissemination of program	Spread of effective program and resultant policy— process evaluation of dissemination	Measures of scale-up including program reach and uptake, adaptation and fidelity

5.5 Summary

This chapter has described some of the challenges in intervention evaluations that generate evidence about effectiveness. First, the selection of people for the program was described. Then the steps of evaluation design, measurement issues and statistical testing are summarised. The better the research methods used, the more confident we can be that the observed effects of a program were caused by the intervention and did not occur by chance or due to other influences. In all evaluation studies, there is an obligation to fully describe potential sources of bias, the sampling methods used and methods of data analysis in any report.

Measurement is a central part of impact evaluation. As well as the obvious impact or outcome measurements, relevant measures and indicators are needed at all stages of evaluation, from problem definition to outcomes assessment. The scope of health promotion measurement has expanded from individual-level assessment of health beliefs and behaviours through to measures of concepts such as social capital, community empowerment and the attributes of coalitions and partnerships. In the latter areas, few measures exist and may need to be developed to assess health promotion actions, organisational or environmental outcomes and community-level social outcomes.

In summary, 'best practice' in health promotion evaluation requires continuous consideration of the optimal evaluation methods against those that are feasible in a particular evaluation. No single approach represents the best evaluation design for all purposes. Often qualitative data is useful to confirm or refute quantitative findings. The best approach will vary depending on the context and setting of the program, the resources and time available, and the expressed needs of stakeholders for evidence of a program. In particular, as health promotion programs are larger and more complex (see Chapter 6), the potential for randomisation of participants and extensive validated assessments may become more limited.

References

Bauman AE, Sallis JF, Dzewaltowski DA, et al. (2002). Towards a better understanding of the influences on physical activity: the role of determinants, correlates, causal variables, mediators, moderators and confounders. American Journal of Preventative Medicine 23(2 Suppl):5–14.

Gumz A, Weigel A, Wegscheider K, et al. (2018). The psychenet public health intervention for anorexia nervosa: a pre–post-evaluation study in a female patient sample. Primary Health Care Research and Development 19(1):42–52.

McConnell D, Breitkreuz R & Savage, A (2012). Independent evaluation of the Triple P Positive Parenting Program in family support service settings. Child and Family Social Work 17(1):43–54.

Ng TP, Feng L, Nyunt MSZ, et al. (2015). Nutritional, physical, cognitive, and combination interventions and frailty reversal among older adults:

a randomized controlled trial. The American Journal of Medicine Nov 1; 128(11):1225–36, e1221.

Omer K, Joga A, Dutse U, et al. (2021). Impact of universal home visits on child health in Bauchi State, Nigeria: a stepped wedge cluster randomised controlled trial. BMC Health Services Research 21(1):1085.

Su SY & Huang JY (2020). Effect of nationwide screening program on colorectal cancer mortality in Taiwan: a controlled interrupted time series analysis. International Journal of Colorectal Disease 35(2): 239–47.

Tudor-Sfetea C, Rabee R, Najim M, et al. (2018). Evaluation of two mobile health apps in the context of smoking cessation: qualitative study of cognitive behavioral therapy (CBT) versus NON-CBT-based digital solutions. JMIR mHealth and uHealth 6(4).

Victor RG, Lynch K, Li N, et al. (2018). A cluster-randomized trial of blood-pressure reduction in black barbershops. New England Journal of Medicine 378(14):1291–301.

Vissenberg C, Nierkens V, Van Valkengoed I, et al. (2017). The impact of a social network based intervention on self-management behaviours among patients with type 2 diabetes living in socioeconomically deprived neighbourhoods: a mixed methods approach. Scandinavian Journal of Public Health 45(6):569–83.

Widmer RJ, Allison TG, Lennon R, et al. (2017). Digital health intervention during cardiac rehabilitation: a randomized controlled trial. American Heart Journal 188:65–72.

Further reading

BMJ statistics series (multiple online BMJ short papers 1996–2018, accessible explanations of statistics, from simple methods to more complex ones). Online: https://www.bmj.com/specialties/statistics-notes

6

Systems approaches and comprehensive (complex) program evaluations

Many 'wicked' problems, such as tobacco and alcohol use and obesity, have multiple and complex causes and require more comprehensive strategies to address these multiple causes. Simple interventions focused on one part of the problem are less likely to produce sustainable changes at scale. Even multi-component programs limited to a single setting may be insufficient to address population-level problems (see Figure 6.1). For example, multi-component interventions to promote healthy eating in schools can have an impact on food consumption among school students on school days but have limited impact on food consumed in the family home and out of school.

Figure 6.1 Comprehensiveness of programs for evaluation

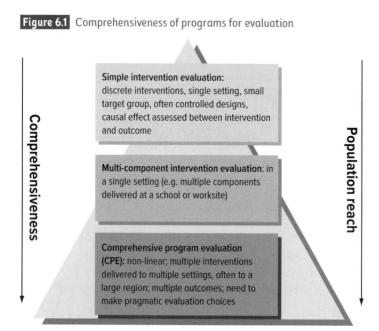

Comprehensiveness

Population reach

Simple intervention evaluation: discrete interventions, single setting, small target group, often controlled designs, causal effect assessed between intervention and outcome

Multi-component intervention evaluation: in a single setting (e.g. multiple components delivered at a school or worksite)

Comprehensive program evaluation (CPE): non-linear; multiple interventions delivered to multiple settings, often to a large region; multiple outcomes; need to make pragmatic evaluation choices

This chapter addresses the challenges in evaluating the comprehensive programs required to address these multifactorial problems.

6.1 Comprehensive public health programs

In these circumstances 'comprehensive' (complex) programs are often needed. For example, past investment in school-based smoking education programs have been shown to be ineffective at influencing smoking among young people in the absence of broader measures to limit tobacco promotion and supply. Any single intervention in a single setting alone is unlikely to solve the problem of childhood obesity, and comprehensive programs of work across multiple settings are needed. Practical experience in designing and implementing such complex programs has evolved over several decades, through the 1986 Ottawa Charter for Health Promotion, the evolution of environment and policy interventions, using the concept of socioecological models to describe population strategies and through to recent development in 'systems thinking'. Evaluation designs and methods for these more complex programs are significantly different to those that might be used for simpler, more focused interventions such as those described in Chapter 5.

6.2 Comprehensive (complex) program evaluation (CPE)

True 'complex (comprehensive) programs' in public health are uncommon. They are comprised of 'several interacting elements aimed at whole populations or community settings ... targeting any or all of individuals, settings, professionals or policy makers' (Craig et al. 2008). Their evaluation requires assessment of a whole program of work, comprised of multiple components in multiple settings, sometimes working across a whole system. For example, a comprehensive national program to reduce cardiovascular disease risk would require interventions and programs delivered across professional groups, health and non-health sectors and across diverse geographic regions.

Comprehensive programs need different approaches to evaluation compared to the single interventions discussed in Chapter 5. These comprehensive approaches require multiple 'evaluations', over a prolonged time frame and across settings, making it difficult to use scientific designs such as randomised trials (Skivington et al. 2021). Further, with the diversity of stakeholders and target groups, it may be difficult to standardise the 'program' that is delivered, and adaptation will occur across settings. These differences also point to the need for more detailed evaluation planning, prioritisation of elements to be evaluated and the mix of quantitative and qualitative methods to be used.

Many aspects of a comprehensive health program are complex, from the planning stages through to the choice of outcome(s). Evaluators need to define the key components in the proposed program of work, and identify the processes and outcomes likely to be influenced by individual components and their combinations. They need to engage multiple stakeholders in the planning and evaluation design, and plan for data collection from the outset. These stages are illustrated in Figure 6.2. From left to right, the planning process starts with community and stakeholder consultation and the development of draft logic models. Next, evidence reviews should inform the 'best practice' program components to be implemented. Population health data may help to identify the target populations and settings where interventions are to be delivered. Consideration of context is important, across settings that may differ in acceptance of the program, or in the facilities and resources to run it as intended. Then attention should focus on developing the evaluation design(s) and measures required to assess the outcomes that are hypothesised to change (right-hand side of Figure 6.2).

6.3 Planning for comprehensive program evaluation

Evaluation planning needs to be *pragmatic,* identifying the components where evaluation is most important, otherwise comprehensive program evaluation (CPE) may become unmanageable or unaffordable. A quick checklist for starting to evaluate comprehensive programs includes consideration of the following (Craig et al. 2008; Skivington et al. 2021):

1. The underpinning theory, and likely components of the comprehensive program of work, although these may evolve over several years
2. An initial, but flexible, logic model, which plans the actions, outputs and outcomes of each component, and describes how each component might be measured, and contribute to, endpoint health gain
3. What pilot (formative) evaluation is required to design and test the components of the program, especially in diverse settings
4. Build the evaluation model for each component, identify essential process (implementation) indicators, and identify qualitative methods that may be needed to understand how and why the program works in different contexts
5. Identify impact and outcome measures and consider how and when data are to be collected; in multi-year comprehensive programs, sufficient time frames should be specified at the outset that may permit change to occur and be measured for each of the outcomes (see Figure 1.3)

Figure 6.2 Complexity at multiple levels in a comprehensive health promotion program

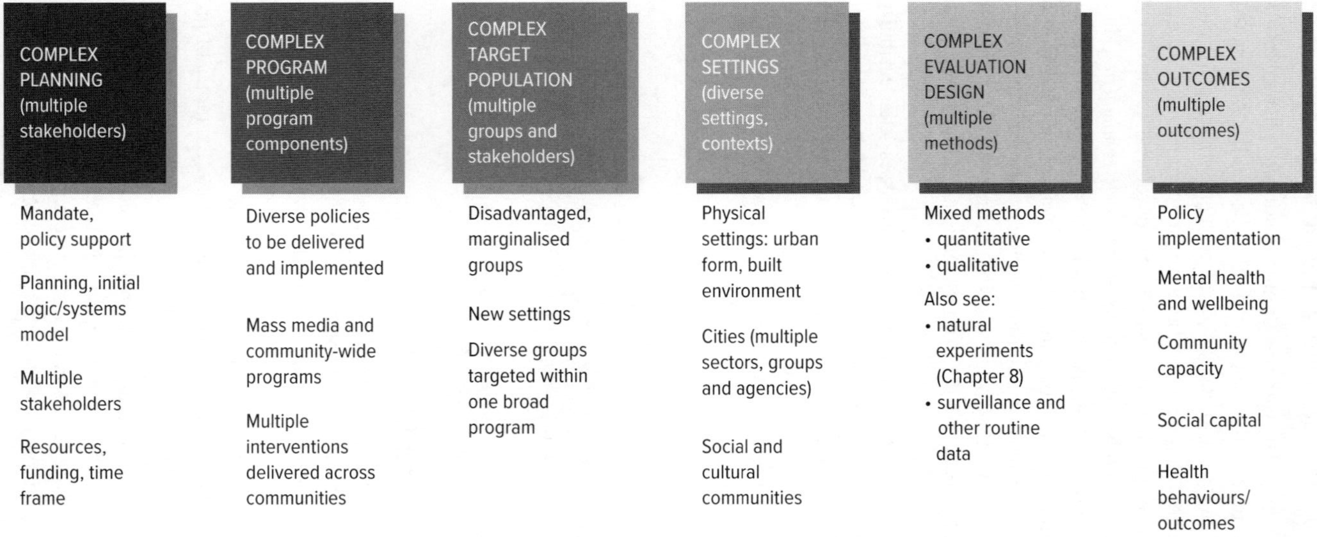

COMPLEX PLANNING (multiple stakeholders)	COMPLEX PROGRAM (multiple program components)	COMPLEX TARGET POPULATION (multiple groups and stakeholders)	COMPLEX SETTINGS (diverse settings, contexts)	COMPLEX EVALUATION DESIGN (multiple methods)	COMPLEX OUTCOMES (multiple outcomes)
Mandate, policy support	Diverse policies to be delivered and implemented	Disadvantaged, marginalised groups	Physical settings: urban form, built environment	Mixed methods • quantitative • qualitative	Policy implementation
Planning, initial logic/systems model	Mass media and community-wide programs	New settings	Cities (multiple sectors, groups and agencies)	Also see: • natural experiments (Chapter 8)	Mental health and wellbeing
Multiple stakeholders	Multiple interventions delivered across communities	Diverse groups targeted within one broad program	Social and cultural communities	• surveillance and other routine data	Community capacity
Resources, funding, time frame					Social capital
					Health behaviours/ outcomes

Formative evaluation for comprehensive programs

Planning for a CPE may start with one or more evidence reviews, stakeholder consultations and the construction of a draft logic model. Although things change in CPEs over time, a baseline and regularly updated logic model provides an updated roadmap for evaluators to continuously inform the project. A detailed evaluation plan should be developed, with objectives, proposed research methods and outcomes *for each component.* The time frames, data collection and measures should be specified at the outset, developed in consultation with stakeholders. For example, considering which of the multiple components of a community injury prevention program need to be pre-tested and how they will be delivered in different contexts, and considering at what time points the primary outcome, injury rates, should be compared with baseline rates.

As with single interventions, it is important to assess the feasibility and costs of implementing a comprehensive program of work; the major difference is the scale and duration, as comprehensive programs usually require the commitment of resources and staffing over several years. Formative evaluation may assess whether the system and the community are primed for the comprehensive program that is being proposed.

> *In the evaluation of comprehensive programs, extensive pre-implementation assessments are essential to confirm that the necessary resources and community and stakeholder engagement is sufficient to support a long-term program of work.*

Process evaluation for CPEs

The central part of CPE is thorough process evaluation, building on the evaluation methods outlined in Chapters 3 to 5. Process evaluation will be required for key components, as well as an overall judgment across the whole program (Moore et al. 2015). Methods are often qualitative, using interviews, focus groups, embedded participant researchers and sometimes case studies to describe program implementation and acceptability. Examples of process evaluation methods include the following.

■ Evaluation of the extent and sustainability of partnerships with stakeholders and the community to drive the changes required in each setting (this can be using quantitative partnership measures, or qualitative interviews with stakeholders, or sometimes, social network analysis).

- Evaluation of the implementation of each component and program reach at multiple levels (intervention fidelity); that is, whether intervention components were delivered as planned and how they varied across different regions and settings (reach, adaptation). These include monitoring the capacity and infrastructure to deliver the program.
- Context; that is, which local and external factors influenced the uptake, delivery and acceptability. This includes realist evaluation using qualitative methods to understand how and whether the program is thought to work, and to answer *what works for whom and in what context?* (Fletcher et al. 2016).
- To determine the degree of adaptation that will still produce useful outcomes. What effects would an intervention have if one or more components was omitted?

As comprehensive programs are the product of multiple parts, it is important to use process evaluation to build an understanding of which components worked, or were delivered well, or were well accepted (or whether they failed). This is instructive to inform future efforts in addressing the same problem. Different qualitative data can be compared against quantitative information collected elsewhere to corroborate or refute evaluation findings; the process known as 'triangulation of data'. These evaluation tasks explain whether the lack of an apparent effect was due to true lack of effect in a population, or to implementation failure (assessed by good process evaluation). Sometimes, process evaluation of comprehensive programs can be further informed by case studies (Fletcher et al. 2016).

Understanding the delivery and implementation mechanisms is important for understanding complex programs and may explain the observed quantitative impact. For this reason, it is essential to carry out high-quality process evaluations in CPE.

Impact/outcome evaluation and research designs for comprehensive programs

Evaluation designs for comprehensive programs employ both qualitative and quantitative methods to carry out multiple parallel and sequential evaluation tasks. Impact evaluation is used to document achievement of the objectives of each program subcomponent. These might include impact measures of changes to community members, school students or workplace employees at a defined baseline and at follow-up, surveys of changes to organisational climate and stakeholders, and assessments of changes made to policy and to social and physical environments. This extends the description of 'health promotion outcomes' presented in Chapter 1 (Figure 1.2), but here multiple outcomes may be concurrently assessed.

Research designs build on those in Chapter 5, with ideal CPEs using randomised or cluster randomised designs (Craig et al. 2008). However, the complexity of real-world interventions (multiple, phased interventions across a whole population) may make a randomised trial design impractical if not impossible (Skivington et al. 2021). Other research designs may be useful; for example, where an intervention involves phased rollout of the intervention across sites (stepped-wedge design), or preference trials, where some degree of choice exists for people to choose a particular intervention component.

A stepped-wedge design may be useful where there is a strong policy interest in implementing a program, but its effectiveness is not known. In some such situations, there may be insufficient resources for the program to be universally provided, so a rollout over time across different regions is proposed, and rollout can occur according to a randomisation schedule (see Chapter 5). Alternatively, quasi-experimental designs are often used, with non-randomly allocated program and comparison regions, and if carefully planned, can provide useful evidence of program effects (Bell et al. 2019; also see Chapter 5).

Summative evaluation of comprehensive programs

In some situations, it may be possible to use existing routinely collected population surveys to evaluate comprehensive programs. This is often in addition to data collected in the evaluation of a comprehensive program, but sometimes these routine population data are the only quantitative estimates of outcomes collected. Population surveys are often conducted annually, and can be used to track health-related changes in the population in a standardised way over the life of the program and provide a summary of its overall effect on specific outcomes. Examples include tracking smoking rates among adolescents or monitoring the number of injurious falls among older adults that occur in a community. Serial population surveys need to have sufficient sample sizes to track changes in the regions of interest and need the flexibility to include survey questions relevant to the CPE.

The summary conclusions of a CPE are sometimes described as *summative evaluation.* This considers data from different sources and collected using diverse methods, and it describes an overall picture of success. The conclusions from different types of data are compared to see if the findings corroborate each other.

For example, consider the potential evaluation components that you might develop to assess an integrated multisite intervention to reduce sun exposure among school-age children.

Formative evaluation

- Was the sun protection program evidence-based with previous research showing its effectiveness?
- Was there piloting of the intervention in different settings, and discussions with key stakeholders about its delivery?
- Was there a budget, timeline and logic model developed to guide the evaluation?

Process evaluation

- How aware are participants of the issue, program and/or message (program exposure)?
- Was the sun protection policy implemented the same way across regions (fidelity and reach, and assessing any adaptation made)?
- Did qualitative interviews with groups of parents from diverse cultural backgrounds indicate that they understood the sun protection messages in the same way?

Impact and outcome evaluations

- Did the school education modules about sun protection have the same impact in different schools?
- Did the mass media campaign targeting parents reach all diverse population groups?
- Did sun protection practices among parents and children and at school level change over time?

Summative evaluation

- This stage considers all the implementation information as well as the different impact and outcome results. If evaluations of separate components point in the same direction (well implemented in schools and communities; school students changed their sun protection practices; different groups of parents aware of the initiative), then the data are concordant, indicating a successful overall or 'summative' evaluation of this comprehensive program.

6.4 Challenges in conducting CPEs

Systems-level evaluation

The community-wide system in which CPEs are used poses challenges to evaluation theory and practice (McGill et al. 2021). Evaluation of systems approaches comprise studies that explore the interrelated factors in the system, or evaluate the processes and impacts of parts or all of the system. For example, evaluating a national COVID-19 immunisation program must consider the diversity of community views and policy priorities regarding the vaccine, vaccine delivery issues, workforce issues and settings for vaccination to occur. Actions in one part of the system may have consequences in other parts of the system. In evaluation terms, understanding the system dynamics can assist in decisions on the nature of evaluation methods and assessing the components that should be monitored.

We propose a pragmatic approach to systems-level CPE evaluation. A researcher-led approach would place greater emphasis on understanding the system; for example, using realist evaluation methods or a greater emphasis on assessing outcomes using controlled designs (which would be expensive to maintain long term). A pragmatic approach assumes that the design and conduct of evaluation are developed to meet the needs of the complex system being evaluated. There needs to be flexibility in the evaluation plan, as implementation may not follow a linear logic model as clearly as in a single-component intervention. In practice, the implementation may be delayed in different parts of a system and may not be implemented universally as planned. Observing, recording and reflecting on these variations in implementation form an essential part of the overall evaluation.

Time to achieve outcomes

Impact and outcome data are often collected, but sufficient time is needed between the multiple components delivered and community changes becoming evident. If documenting program impact is considered achievable, or is politically necessary, then it is important to consider the research design and the choice of outcomes that might be achieved in the time required. However, caution must be exercised in expecting short-term results from comprehensive programs. Timescales measured in years may be necessary for assessing the effects of multiple intervention components across a whole population (see Figure 1.3).

This is particularly true where a systems approach is used. It is challenging to implement and sustain complex programs of work for long enough to achieve demonstrable community-changing effects, so evaluation metrics must be tailored to those that are achievable in specified time frames. Further, there may be concurrent programs or policies at work in parts of the system addressing the same health issue, and it may not be possible to disentangle the causal contributions of individual components. The evaluation of these programs may also benefit from assessment of the partnerships or networks required to optimise the system.

Beyond individual change

The intersecting elements of a comprehensive program target change at these different levels, and the challenge in evaluation is to measure more than just individual-level change. The research design and measurement tasks summate to a set of mixed methods subevaluations within the overall CPE. Evaluation measures may include changes to policies, organisations, delivery systems or community services. Finally, collecting information on program costs and calculating cost-effectiveness may be useful in deciding if a comprehensive approach is worthwhile, as these are long-term, large-scale investments in public health and require substantial resources and commitment.

6.5 Examples of CPEs

Good examples of CPE show the best possible scientific rigour in impact evaluation, and a range of appropriate and often mixed methods across formative and process evaluation components, in order to understand the program's results and explain why and where an intervention component worked or did not work, which is important for subsequent CPE efforts in this area. Three examples are shown in Table 6.1. The first example targets adolescent health and resilience and illustrates the systems approach to evaluation (Rosas & Knight 2019). The Well London project (Phillips et al. 2014) addresses the evaluation components in a program targeting social

Table 6.1 Published examples of CPEs showing complexity in formative, process and impact evaluation

Author (year) and project	Formative evaluation (FE) and process evaluation (PE)	Impact evaluation/ intervention design	Issues around complexity
Rosas & Knight (2019): systems approach to adolescent resilience in three communities in Delaware, United States	Informed by logic model development and 2 years' detailed system mapping activity; used complexity science to identify intervention components and evaluation methods	Steps in evaluation: Group/stakeholder analyses; systems mapping Impact assessed through network analysis changes, changes in collaborative relationships	Showed how systems approaches can be used for complex health promotion programs; however, given issue complexity and community differences, had not yet reached outcome evaluation after 7–8 years

(Continued)

Table 6.1 *Continued*

Author (year) and project	Formative evaluation (FE) and process evaluation (PE)	Impact evaluation/ intervention design	Issues around complexity
Phillips et al. (2014): comprehensive program targets disadvantaged communities in London, United Kingdom	Fourteen projects, each with own process evaluation; mostly mixed methods used; clear positive reported effects in community interviews	Cluster RCT (20 intervention and 20 control communities) on multiple outcomes at 3.5 years follow-up; no significant effects on primary health, wellbeing or social outcomes	Change seen in some subprojects; dose–response— more program exposure seems beneficial; qualitative and quantitative results differed; follow-up may be too soon to see results
Bell et al. (2019): OPAL 9-year project to prevent childhood obesity in South Australia; multi-component systems approach	Multiple process evaluation studies; positive effects on stakeholders and increased community leadership	Quasi-experimental study of primary school students in 20 intervention and 20 matched comparison communities; follow-up 2–3 years	Impact/outcomes: no change in healthy weight between groups (although trends favoured intervention); most other outcomes also showed non-significant differences

Lists of additional papers from these studies presented on the companion Evaluation website: https://evaluationinanutshell.com/

disadvantage and wellbeing in British communities. (Also see http://www. welllondon. org.uk/1145/research-evaluation.html.) The third example, Obesity Prevention and Lifestyle (OPAL), addresses childhood obesity prevention (Bell et al. 2019). The second and third projects illustrate program and evaluation complexity, with inconsistent findings sometimes reported between qualitative and quantitative research results.

6.6 Summary

Single-component interventions may be insufficient to address the myriad determinants of public health problems, and a multilayered program of work over a longer time period is required. Comprehensive programs, comprised of multiple components delivered at different levels, may be needed to tackle these 'wicked' problems. These need evaluation of multiple elements, using mixed qualitative and quantitative techniques, and a summative evaluation at the end of the program. These are long-term, resource-intensive programs, and evaluation efforts need to be equally sophisticated, using high-quality process and impact evaluation to assess complex programs. The mix of quality evaluation and pragmatism is applied to evaluate these programs; this leads to the best scientific rigour possible, as well as qualitative information from participants, stakeholders and program delivery staff to identify reasons for program success and failure. The science and art of CPE necessitates substantial multidisciplinary evaluation expertise and resources.

References

Bell L, Ullah S, Leslie E, et al. (2019). Changes in weight status, quality of life and behaviours of South Australian primary school children: results from the Obesity Prevention and Lifestyle (OPAL) community intervention program. BMC Public Health 19(1):1–14.

Craig P, Dieppe P, Macintyre S, et al. (2008). Developing and evaluating complex interventions: the new MRC Guidance. BMJ 29 September; 337:a1655.

Fletcher A, Jamal F, Moore G, et al. (2016). Realist complex intervention science: applying realist principles across all phases of the Medical Research Council framework for developing and evaluating complex interventions. Evaluation 22(3):286–303.

McGill E, Penney T, Egan M, et al. (2021). Evaluation of public health interventions from a complex systems perspective: a research methods review. Social Science & Medicine 1;272:113697.

Moore GF, Audrey S, Barker M, et al. (2015). Process evaluation of complex interventions: Medical Research Council guidance. BMJ (Online) 19:350.

Phillips G, Bottomley C, Schmidt E, et al. (2014). Well London Phase-1: results among adults of a cluster-randomised trial of a community engagement approach to improving health behaviours and mental well-being in deprived inner-city neighbourhoods. Journal of Epidemiology and Community Health 68(7):606–14.

Rosas S & Knight E (2019). Evaluating a complex health promotion intervention: case application of three systems methods. Critical Public Health 29(3):337–52.

Skivington K, Matthews L, Simpson SA, et al. (2021). Framework for the development and evaluation of complex interventions: gap analysis, workshop and consultation-informed update. Health Technology Assessment 25(57):1–132.

7

Evaluation methods for program replication, scale-up (dissemination) and institutionalisation

Public health change requires reaching large proportions of the population with an intervention. This chapter is concerned with evaluation of efforts to test established interventions in new groups (replication studies) and to scale them up to even larger populations (scale-up or dissemination). This generally requires increasing the emphasis on process evaluation to understand how implementation of interventions work at a larger scale.

This chapter builds on Chapters 5 and 6, which described the evaluation of individual and comprehensive public health interventions, and is concerned with the stages of program replication, scale-up and institutionalisation, beyond the initial testing of whether a program works. These stages of replication, scale-up and institutionalisation are based on the need to deliver interventions and programs to larger and more representative groups. These are illustrated as stages 4, 5 and 6 in Figure 7.1 (which adds to Figure 2.1 in Chapter 2).

Health promotion interventions found to be effective, affordable and consistently capable of implementation are most likely to attract the attention of funders as suitable for policy support, scale-up and even institutionalisation. It is unwise to base a policy decision to scale-up a program and commit significant funding on evidence that is derived from one evaluation study, especially if results are equivocal or the effects are small. This is true even if the issue is a key priority, but evidence of successful interventions is scarce.

The results of negative evaluations are also important, but often ignored; programs shown repeatedly not to be effective should not be considered for dissemination.

7.1 Stages in assessing the significance of programs

This chapter describes the three stages of replication, scale-up (dissemination) and institutionalisation. Across these stages, increasing numbers in the target population are exposed to and engage with the intervention. The three stages may seem obvious, but after years of working on solutions to public health problems, practitioners and researchers may lose sight of the population-wide goal represented by these stages. Put simply, policymakers and practitioners need more practice-relevant 'evidence' on interventions feasible for implementation at scale within available (constrained) resources and service configurations. Providing this evidence requires testing scaled-up program delivery using different evaluation methods to those typically used in researcher-led efficacy studies described in Chapter 5.

The model in Chapter 2 is re-drawn here as Figure 7.1 to identify the practitioner challenges in evaluating scale-up (demonstration, scale-up and intervention monitoring) and the researcher's role in implementation science. Note that the third row of Figure 7.1 with light shading focuses on the role of implementation science, which is the purview of researchers, and is explained later in this chapter (see Box 7.1). The last row focuses on translational policy actions and scale-up, which is work carried out in the health promotion practice system and by policymakers. This shows how thinking about scale-up can occur early, before and during studies of efficacy and effectiveness testing. This can influence the kinds of efficacy studies tested, and their feasibility for scale-up, with the resources consumed and community acceptability considered even during the scientific study that identifies if the intervention works. Subsequently, in stages 4 to 6, the translational work is often carried out by policymakers, assessing the fit of evidence-based interventions in real-world settings.

The differences between those that are researcher-initiated and those that are policymaker's actions in replication and scale-up are further illustrated in Figure 7.2. This mirrors the stages of public health program evaluation in Chapter 2, and in Figure 7.1. The left-hand side of Figure 7.2 shows 'researcher-driven' evaluation tasks that generally reflect research funding opportunities. These entail the application of research methods to produce high-quality scientific evaluation of efficacy, and eventual publication in the scientific literature. There may be a cycle of refining and testing alternative interventions (e.g. using different behaviour change approaches in the same setting), but again these are usually repeated in small-scale or selected samples. Note that implementation science researchers also have a role later in the stages of evaluation, through the scientific testing of different approaches to scaling-up, shown in the dotted arrow in the lower part of the diagram.

Figure 7.1 Stages of public health program evaluation with a focus on scale-up and implementation

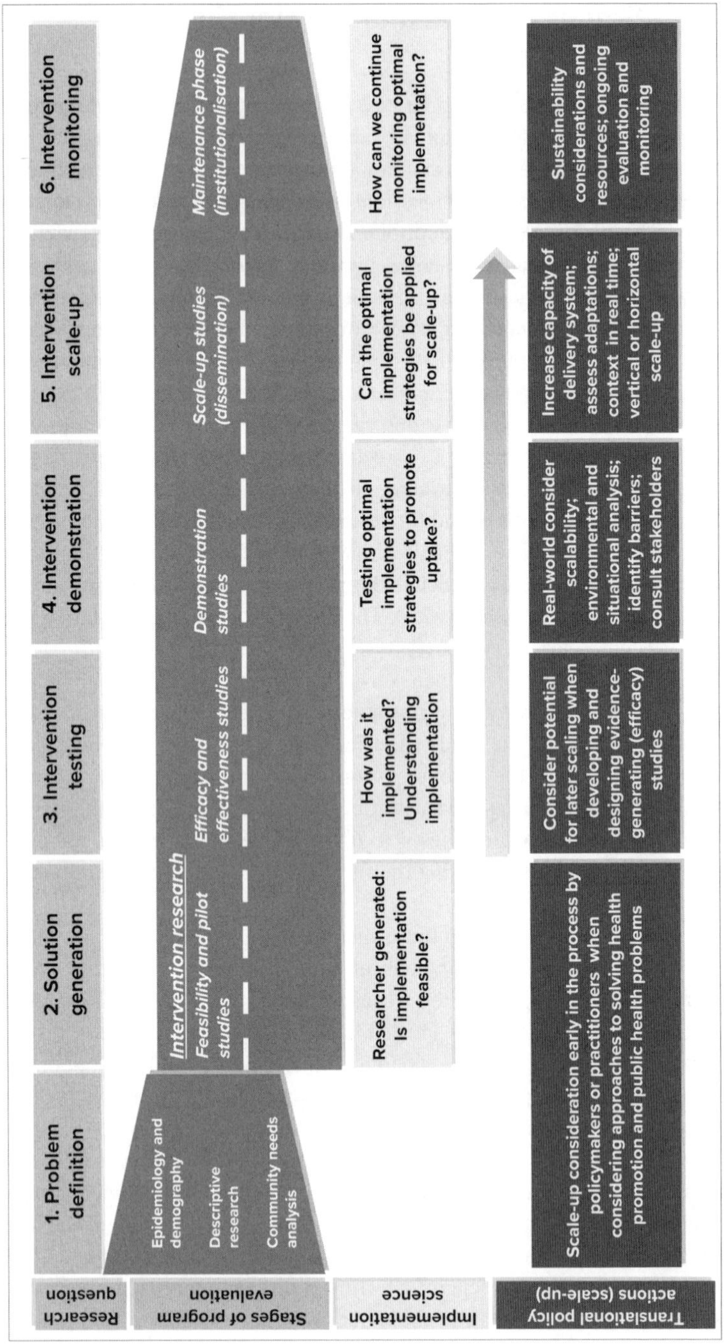

The right-hand side of Figure 7.2 shows the practitioner interest in evaluation of the replication and scale-up stages. Given the health promotion priorities and resources in a particular region, consideration will be given to the evidence being generated by researchers on the left-hand side of the figure. If circumstances support the need and capacity for population-wide reach of specific evidence-based programs, then the process of 'research translation' begins. This is comprised of testing interventions and programs in new settings and with new populations and disseminated to whole regions, or in ways that can be adopted at a system level and institutionalised in public health practice. This 'research translation' process is usually led by government departments or non-government organisations (NGOs), or occasionally the private sector, and the evaluation methods are different, with an emphasis on process evaluation (to assess implementation) of the efficacious interventions generated on the left-hand side of the figure.

Figure 7.2 Researcher and policymaker roles in replication and scale-up (dissemination)

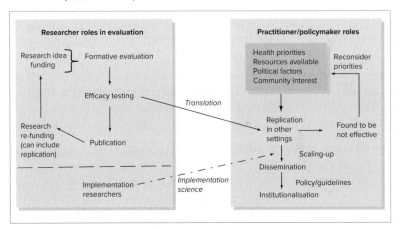

7.2 Evaluation methods in replication studies (intervention demonstration)

Replication or intervention demonstration is the testing of a successful intervention in new settings and circumstances to demonstrate implementation challenges and assess if the effects of the original efficacy trial are maintained. Often, efficacy studies will rely on motivated frontline workers (clinicians, schoolteachers) and may attract socially and educationally advantaged participants with high levels of health literacy. Replicating the intervention allows us to develop confidence in the generalisability of the findings to other groups and settings, and to understand the practical aspects of implementing a program in different environments and contexts—providing the basis for subsequent scale-up.

Replication increases confidence that the effects observed from an efficacy study might be achieved with different populations in different circumstances. The more replication of this (or very similar) interventions, the more confidence you can have in the findings and the better placed you will be to make subsequent decisions on whether to scale-up an intervention.

Evaluation methods for replication are different to those in the initial efficacy study. It is important that replication studies use identical outcome measures, so that effects are comparable. The evaluation designs for replication studies might use designs described in Chapter 5, such as quasi-experimental or controlled trials, but could utilise 'before–after' designs. The latter design may be acceptable in replication studies because the effect size is already established from the original efficacy trial. The settings chosen are not necessarily randomly sampled; in replication studies purposive sampling can maximise the diversity of settings in which to test the intervention.

Conducting good process evaluation is central to replication studies. We need to identify if the program can be implemented as intended in different settings, or whether it will require adaptation. These contextual differences may be due to different levels of resourcing and management support or different characteristics of program participants. This information is essential for health practitioners responsible for implementing programs.

If the program implementation cannot be replicated (with adaptation as necessary) in different circumstances, then further implementation of the program in different sites would not be likely to yield the same results as the original program.

Process evaluation in the replication phase also helps to identify effective mechanisms for conducting the intervention in different groups and settings. Examples are shown in Table 7.1. The first study listed replicates a mental health literacy program among university students in the United Kingdom; however, the antecedent evidence was a post-only evaluation conducted in Canada, suggesting that critical appraisal of reported evidence is needed. The second example is a community replication of clinical lifestyle programs and shows positive effects using a randomised trial. The third example shows Canadian programs to increase physical activity among older adults, with initial testing in diverse settings, prior to scale-up.

Table 7.1 Replication and scale-up (dissemination) examples*

Author (year)	Intervention	Replication/scale-up
Replication studies		
Hunt, Wei & Kutcher (2019)	Mental health literacy training	Repeated in a United Kingdom university sample, with some positive effects
Bartels et al. (2015)	Mental health problems and overweight—evidence generated in clinical settings	Replicated in community setting, controlled trial, significant effects shown
McKay et al. (2018)	Older adults' quality of life; assessing whether the effects are similar in different contexts	Choose to Move, evidence-based older adults physical activity program, tested in multiple community sites
Scale-up studies		
Hunt et al. (2020)	Football fans in training—lifestyle program for middle-aged men; existing initial efficacy and effectiveness studies	Mapped against scale-up criteria, documented scale-up and maintained delivery
McKay et al. (2015)	Action Schools! BC implementation—primary school health promotion	Illustrates stages from efficacy to effectiveness to province-wide scale-up
Lam et al. (2019)	Evidence base (trials) that oral rehydration salts (ORS) and zinc treat diarrhoea in preschool children	Scale-up to three provinces in India, effects protective at scale
Implementation trials (implementation science)		
Chinman et al. (2018)	Implementation as primary outcome; but this is also replication, as it tests the same intervention method used for effective teen pregnancy prevention	Assessed in cluster randomised controlled trial (RCT) design, testing different implementation approaches to alcohol prevention

*Additional examples can be found on the companion Evaluation website: https://evaluationinanutshell.com/

Replication studies are not funded as often as efficacy trials because the need for this stage is not always clear to academic research funders or policymakers. Frustratingly, evidence generated from efficacy studies is often used by policymakers as sufficient for widespread dissemination.

Without an understanding of the implementation challenges faced in 'real-world' conditions, a program is less likely to be successfully scaled-up and less likely to produce the intended outcomes when disseminated widely.

7.3 Evaluation methods for scale-up (dissemination)

If a program can be successfully replicated, it can be considered for wider scale-up across systems or regions. Dissemination (or scale-up) is an intentional process to reach more people across a population or region. It is defined as the process of 'achieving the maximum uptake of effective and feasible interventions into a community' (World Health Organization [WHO] 2010). 'Scale-up' can be pursued in two different ways. 'Horizontal' scale-up occurs when an intervention is disseminated through services and settings to reach an increasing proportion of a population. 'Vertical' scale-up occurs when a program is disseminated through government policy so that the policy is widely taken up, ideally in circumstances where previous efficacy and replication studies have indicated the need for continuing commitment and resources from decision-makers and funders.

Milat and colleagues (2016) and others have described several stages that typically occur from initiation through to delivering an intervention at scale (WHO 2010). These stages have many similarities to the planning models describer earlier in Chapter 1 and can be summarised as follows.

1. *Initial steps:* Clarification of the alignment of the intervention with current public (government and community) priorities. This is different to researcher-initiated evaluations, which are based on scientific testing of theoretical or conceptual models for change. The initial steps for scale-up are to review evidence for efficacy and any replication of the intervention in other settings, and identification of any informative research syntheses.

2. *Planning for scale-up:* The planning stage for scale-up has some similarities with planning for efficacy, in that an initial logic model describing the core components of the intervention is needed. However, the first difference is consideration of scalability: are the time and conditions and the health promotion system suitable for research translation? Other differences include consideration of diverse contexts and environments, the mobilisation of stakeholders and delivery systems, the identification of realistic resources and consideration of realistic timeframes (O'Hara et al. 2014).

3. *Prepare for scale-up:* This is the formative evaluation stage of scale-up, comprising consultation with stakeholders and the work of engaging with and building capacity in the system/workforce that will deliver the

intervention across contexts and settings. Testing of the intervention in different settings is needed, and discussion regarding feasibility held with local delivery agents, especially if the stage of intervention demonstration has not been fully completed.

4. *Delivery at scale:* The evaluation tasks are: defining the important process evaluation indicators that should be measured (implementation); monitoring the organisations and agents who will deliver the program; and assessing to what degree and when outcomes will be measured.

5. *Consider sustainability:* Plan for sustainment at scale, identify longer term delivery system options and resources, and identify ongoing ownership of the program to ensure maintenance across contexts.

These stages indicate that the tasks for planning and evaluating at scale are different to those required for earlier stages of evidence generation and replication. These stages will differ when considering secondary prevention (scale-up in clinical settings) compared to population scale-up. In clinical settings, there is a greater consistency of setting (health services and the health system), with the delivery agents usually healthcare providers. This may be more straightforward to implement, compared to community and population settings, where partnerships and engagement for scale-up are needed with a range of diverse groups as well as with community members.

Consideration of scale-up should ideally begin as the efficacy studies are designed. For example, an efficacy study should consider from the outset whether the costs, complexity and intensity of an intervention could be reproduced in different circumstances if the intervention is demonstrated to be effective. The importance of formative and process evaluation is heightened in assessing the feasibility of scale-up (O'Hara et al. 2014). Reflective tools are available for practitioners considering whether an intervention of proven effectiveness can be easily scaled-up, such as the Intervention Scalability Assessment Tool (Milat et al. 2020).

It is also important to recognise that decisions to scale-up do not occur in a vacuum and will most likely be supported in the confluence of policy, resources and priorities and the existence of evidence-based interventions, known as the opportunistic 'scale-up window'. The best efforts at scale-up will have demonstrable leadership, a clear mandate and resources, a timeframe, good partnerships with stakeholders and clear links to policy priorities. It is important to retain focus on the best evaluation methods possible when faced with imperatives to scale-up quickly, or to attempt to address population-wide dissemination of a program with insufficient resources. Thus, pragmatic decisions about which elements to evaluate become important; it may be necessary to collect good information on only a subset of process or outcome indicators, or to assess reach and uptake in a sample of regions which have received the program.

Examples of scale-up evaluation methods and measures are shown in Table 7.2. The three examples indicate the full series of stages moving from efficacy to effectiveness to scale-up (McKay et al. 2015; Hunt et al. 2020) and illustrate the evaluation of delivery at scale (Lam et al. 2019). Scale-up evaluation will vary across different 'systems', dependent on their complexity and the extent to which systems-level evaluation is needed (see Chapter 6). The research designs will also vary, but the emphasis on process evaluation suggests that pragmatic evaluations of scale-up in the real world will often utilise quasi-experimental or before–after designs.

A systems approach, involving the interaction of interventions, processes and settings, requires more flexible evaluation methods across the relevant sets of environments in delivery at scale.

Table 7.2 Evaluation methods and measures for scale-up (dissemination)

Formative evaluation measures	Co-planning for scale-up with practitioners; assessing scalability (Milat et al. 2020); formative evaluation with stakeholders and communities to assess feasibility of, and methods for, program delivery at scale
Process evaluation	Process evaluation indicators and measures including: context, scale-up feasibility; community and stakeholder acceptability and support; program delivery systems and program adaptation; appropriateness of the program across contexts; satisfaction with the program; and presence of suitable community infrastructure and environments
	Workforce capacity, delivery system, resources, champions/advocates for the program
	In addition, explanatory research is sometimes conducted to assess why and how the program worked in different contexts, often using qualitative methods
Impact/outcomes	Focus on process measures, but may measure impact to assess that delivery at scale produces similar effects to efficacy/replication studies; often tested using 'before–after' designs, as effect size should be already known from previous research
Costs	Economic evaluation at scale; document inputs; costs of staffing, delivery, program infrastructure and resources costs; number of people who are reached by and engage with the program

This book provides a pragmatic approach, where the drivers and funders of scale-up are usually in government and occasionally the non-government or private sectors. Sufficient capacity and resources are needed to scale-up and maintain public health programs, beyond the scope of researcher-initiated projects. However, researchers contribute through the application of implementation science, which answers researcher-initiated questions to better understand and optimise intervention implementation. Implementation science is summarised in Box 7.1. The tasks of implementation scientists in the stages of evaluation were shown earlier in Figure 7.1.

BOX 7.1: Implementation science

Implementation is a routine part of process evaluation of any program (see Chapters 2 and 4). Implementation *science* is a subset of implementation work usually controlled by research investigators. It comprises the research methods used to understand, inform and improve implementation practice (Curran et al. 2012). Implementation science is shown in Figure 7.1, and in Figure 7.2 across the stages of program evaluation. The kinds of projects undertaken by implementation scientists include explanatory studies of factors influencing implementation and rigorous studies to assess the effectiveness of different implementation strategies to maximise program uptake. These studies, known as implementation trials, are often characterised as type 1 (studies to assess program efficacy but that also consider implementation and process evaluation), type 2 hybrid-effectiveness implementation studies (test both efficacy and implementation) and type 3 (test implementation strategies for known efficacious programs) (Curran et al. 2012). Other implementation scientists focus on understanding the mechanisms of program action or reach, often using qualitative methods, including stakeholder and end-user analyses and realist evaluation methods.

Implementation science can answer questions more scientifically, but this takes time. This may contrast with the acute needs of policymakers, where evaluation needs are immediate in relation to the proposed program scale-up. There is clear overlap between implementation scientists and the pragmatic work of evaluating scaled-up interventions, but the latter are often embedded in practice, and evaluation is supported by policymakers, whereas implementation science is led by researchers, with resources provided by research funding agencies (see Figure 7.2 and Table 2.1).

7.4 Evaluation methods for the stage of institutionalisation

The last stage in the program evaluation process (stage 6 in Figure 7.1 and Figure 2.1) concerns the monitoring of a program that has been widely disseminated and has become part of routine public health service delivery. This stage of institutionalisation is primarily concerned with quality control and long-term monitoring and surveillance of outcomes at a population level. Institutionalised programs are accepted as needed across the population, delivered over many years and sustained by the public health or other systems. Few published examples exist, as this stage reflects the routine practices of public health agencies. Examples might include established 'Quitlines' offering telephone-based tobacco cessation counselling, mandated school-entry immunisation programs and established routine cancer screening programs.

Assessing and monitoring successful institutionalisation may involve:

■ regular service delivery monitoring or routine population health surveys to assess maintenance of the specific program components (e.g. sustained policy implementation, provision of universal screening tests and individual behaviour change); this includes an equity focus to ensure that all population subgroups can and are accessing the intervention

■ monitoring continuing community engagement and support for the intervention

■ quality control (process evaluation) to confirm that the established program is consistently delivered as intended

■ continually considering the relationship between the costs of a scale-up program and its population health benefits.

Process evaluation remains central to institutionalisation and will require dedicated resources. Implementation across many sites requires quality control to make sure that the programs delivered have enough elements of the original program to remain effective. These routine evaluation tasks can assist frontline workers, managers and policymakers to support the ongoing maintenance of established programs.

7.5 Summary

This chapter has focused on the different evaluation tasks and measures for the replication, scale-up and institutionalisation of health promotion programs. These are the stages of program evaluation with an increasing population focus, as shown in Figure 7.1.

Once an intervention has been demonstrated to be effective, it should be replicated in other settings and, if it maintains effectiveness in different environments, it should then be scaled-up. In these latter stages, the central component is process evaluation, often using qualitative research methods, ensuring that the program is delivered across a community in ways likely to maintain effectiveness. Finally, as programs become institutionalised, population surveys can be used to track outcomes and system quality control measures used across larger regions or national program rollout.

These evaluations inform policymakers of the real-world potential for innovative public health interventions. However, no single approach represents the 'best' evaluation design for all replication and scale-up purposes. One overarching principle is that the evaluation design and methods should be well described in all evaluations, at all stages of intervention testing and dissemination.

References

Bartels SJ, Pratt SI, Aschbrenner KA, et al. (2015). Pragmatic replication trial of health promotion coaching for obesity in serious mental illness and maintenance of outcomes. American Journal of Psychiatry 172(4):344–52.

Chinman M, Ebener P, Malone PS, et al. (2018). Testing implementation support for evidence-based programs in community settings: a replication cluster-randomized trial of Getting To Outcomes®. Implementation Science 13(1).

Curran GM, Bauer M, Mittman B, et al. (2012). Effectiveness-implementation hybrid designs: combining elements of clinical effectiveness and implementation research to enhance public health impact. Medical Care 50(3):217–26.

Hunt S, Wei Y & Kutcher S (2019). Addressing mental health literacy in a UK university campus population: positive replication of a Canadian intervention. Health Education Journal 78(5):537–44.

Hunt K, Wyke S, Bunn C, et al. (2020). Scale-up and scale-out of a gender-sensitized weight management and healthy living program delivered to overweight men via professional sports clubs: the wider implementation of Football Fans in Training (FFIT). International Journal of Environmental Research and Public Health 17(2):584.

Lam F, Pro G, Agrawal S, et al. (2019). Effect of enhanced detailing and mass media on community use of oral rehydration salts and zinc during a scale-up program in Gujarat and Uttar Pradesh. Journal of Global Health 9(1):01501.

McKay HA, Macdonald HM, Nettlefold L, et al. (2015). Action Schools!
BC implementation: from efficacy to effectiveness to scale-up. British
Journal of Sports Medicine 49(4):210–18.

McKay H, Nettlefold L, Bauman A, et al. (2018). Implementation of a
co-designed physical activity program for older adults: positive impact
when delivered at scale. BMC Public Health 18(1):1–5.

Milat AJ, Newson R, King L, et al. (2016). A guide to scaling up population
health interventions. Public Health Research & Practice 26(1):e261104.
Online access to the original report: https://www.health.nsw.gov.au/
research/Pages/scalability-guide.aspx

Milat A, Lee K, Conte K, et al. (2020). Intervention Scalability Assessment
Tool: a decision support tool for health policy makers and implementers.
Health Research Policy and Systems 18(1):1–7.

O'Hara BJ, Phongsavan P, King L, et al. (2014). Translational formative
evaluation: critical in up-scaling public health programmes. Health
Promotion International 29(1):38–46.

World Health Organization (2010). World Health Organization: Nine steps
for developing a scaling-up strategy. WHO. Online: https://apps.who.int
/iris/handle/10665/44432

Further reading

Brownson RC, Colditz GA & Proctor EK (eds) (2012). Dissemination and
Implementation Research in Health: Translating Science to Practice.
Oxford University Press, New York, NY.

Rychetnik L, Bauman A, Laws R, et al. (2012). Translating research for
evidence-based public health: key concepts and future directions. Journal
of Epidemiology and Community Health 66(12):1187–92.

8

Natural experiments: one method of policy evaluation

Health-promoting programs and policies are often introduced universally across a population in a way that significantly limits our ability to apply the type of experimental research designs described in previous chapters. In these circumstances we can still undertake an evaluation using modified methods. This type of evaluation is often referred to as a 'natural experiment' (NE).

8.1 Introduction and rationale

The United Kingdom's Medical Research Council describes NEs as evaluations of health or other outcomes where 'exposure to the event of intention of interest has not been manipulated by the researcher' (Craig et al. 2012). The key issue here is the researcher or evaluator has no control over any aspect of the intervention. Examples might include policies, laws and regulations that have been introduced by government and are applied universally (e.g. a ban on smoking in public places, a tax on sugar-sweetened beverages or mandatory childhood immunisation). Such policies can be generated and implemented by any government department and/or a non-government organisation. Health responses and outcomes from unanticipated natural events and disasters (e.g. earthquakes or floods) and communicable disease outbreaks (e.g. COVID-19) can also be examined as NEs.

NEs are useful where evaluation data are important to inform decision-makers or provide new evidence about intervention effects or health outcomes in circumstances where such information does not already exist. These evaluations are significantly different to those described in the previous chapters because researchers had no part in the design and implementation of policies or programs, but post hoc, develop methods to assess them. Such evaluations can assess (to the extent possible) variations in exposure to the effects of policies and programs, and their subsequent health outcomes. However, although they are a useful addition to evaluation methods, it should be noted that not all policy evaluations require NE methods (see Box 8.1).

The methods and data sources for NEs need to be considered and developed on a case-by-case basis. Evaluation in these circumstances most often focus on observing post-intervention variations in exposure, impact and outcomes between different geographical areas or population groups over time. Most often these NEs rely on routinely available data from existing public sources including, for example, regular health surveys and health services activity. Such routine information and data collections can be assessed prior to the occurrence of the major event or introduction of a policy, and compared to the post-event period, usually using time series designs. NEs may also involve post-implementation data collection on public response to policies and programs. All these data can be used to assess the reach and impact of, for example, new health policies or changes to health service delivery or organisation. Through systematic observation and contextual analysis, it is feasible to examine variation in outcomes and consider critically whether any changes observed are attributable to the intervention or policy.

BOX 8.1: Policy evaluation

There are many kinds of policy and many researchers in multiple disciplines that consider policy analysis, the context and nature of policy, and the theory of change. In addition, policy scientists or researchers consider the processes that lead to policy development and policy formulation, which we would describe as the formative parts of policy evaluation. They are beyond the scope of this text, where we focus on policy implementation and policy impact evaluation as the key features that can be assessed using NEs. Implementation is the process evaluation of whether the policy is rolled out as intended and whether there is variation in different contexts in the uptake or adherence to the policy. Impact or outcome evaluations are assessing the effects of the policy, which may be implemented using complex program evaluation methods or as part of a system (see Chapter 6). This can be the evaluation of government or other regulatory, policy or other rules or regulations related to the environment or other settings.

8.2 Circumstances in which NEs are used

The opportunities for NEs are diverse. The majority emerge in response to the introduction of new public policy and related programs and a desire to assess their effects. Examples include policies such as advertising bans, food regulation, change in taxes to products such as tobacco and alcohol, trade policies, smoking restrictions or gun control legislation. Policies that are not wholly directed at improving health that, for example, support change in the physical environment, built infrastructure, green space developments, transport systems and/or improving urban access can also influence health service utilisation, physical activity or community wellbeing. Many of these policy decisions are outside the influence of the health sector and have their origins in different parts of government. Especially in low- to middle-income countries, NEs can support and inform efforts to control infectious diseases, childhood diseases and maternal health.

A range of NEs are listed in Table 8.1. All examples illustrate the diversity of policy implementation or natural phenomena that are well beyond the influence of researchers. Hence the designs and methods used for NEs are tailored to answer each question differently. These examples illustrate natural experiment evaluations of the impact of policy and policy-informing research, and also sometimes provide new information about the causes of health problems.

Other annotated examples are updated regularly on the companion Evaluation website (https://evaluationinanutshell.com/) and also described in the Scottish Government report (n.d.).

Table 8.1 Examples of natural experiments (NEs)

Author (year) and type of NE	Purpose/design of NE
Islam et al. (2020)	
Policy evaluation NE meta-analysis	Examination of physical distancing interventions and risk of COVID-19 in 149 countries; demonstrated social distancing, school and work closures and early lockdown policies reduced Covid cases [policy-relevant information]
Anyanwu et al. (2020)	
Policy evaluation NE using routine data	Routine data, UK household surveys 1994–2016 showed smoking initiation in adolescents fell after an implementation of smoke-free policy; also reduced inequalities in the distribution of youth smoking
Ejlerskov et al. (2018)	
Policy evaluation NE with comparison region	Some UK supermarkets implemented policy to not display unhealthy foods at the checkout, all other supermarkets as controls. Time series data, initial and 12 month sustained significant reduction in unhealthy food purchases

(Continued)

Table 8.1 *Continued*

Author (year) and type of NE	Purpose/design of NE
Moore et al. (2020)	
Policy evaluation NE	Qualitative and quantitative evaluation (mixed methods) before and after regulations introduced to regulate e-cigarettes—showing role of qualitative methods to corroborate quantitative findings
Fuller et al. (2019)	
Natural event NE	Public transport strike in Philadelphia associated with a 57% increase in public bicycle scheme usage; returned to baseline when strike was over
Sato et al. (2020)	
Natural disaster NE	Association between earthquake and social capital and mental health in serial surveys from a cohort study sample in Japan. Changes in social capital following the earthquake associated with increased depression
Liyanage et al. (2021)	
NE to understand disease causation	Impact of COVID-19 on dengue fever transmission—during COVID-19, reduction in dengue cases in Sri Lanka, demonstrating decreased population mobility reduces dengue risk

8.3 Evaluation methods to assess NEs

There are several issues unique to NE evaluation designs. First, although they can be prospective (if a known policy or event is anticipated), they are usually concurrently or retrospectively evaluated. For example, an event may have already occurred, even in the remote past, but routine data can be monitored prior to and following the event, using time series designs. This methodology can be applied to assess the impact of a policy some time (possibly years) after its implementation provided relevant data have been collected continuously throughout the period.

Substantial technical discussions have occurred regarding designs that could be used in evaluating NEs. We have already discussed pre–post designs, and these can be strengthened in circumstances where a policy or related program is only implemented in one region of a country, allowing for the examination of effects in comparison regions or groups that are not exposed to the policy or program. This design can be further strengthened by using data collected at multiple time points before and after exposure to the policy or program where such data exist. The evaluation of some NEs is based on mixed methods, with qualitative methods (such as interviews with stakeholders or affected communities) used to triangulate data available from other sources. New methods of modelling are also being developed and applied to improve confidence in observed outcomes from NEs, including statistical regression techniques, propensity analysis (a method to approximate exposed and non-exposed groups as if they were from a controlled trial) and the use of synthetic controls (modelling of what would be expected to happen in the absence of a policy or natural phenomenon; Craig et al. 2017).

Quite commonly, natural experiments can have non-randomly allocated comparison regions or control groups, but then fit into a quasi-experimental design. The most common design is probably interrupted time series where routine data are collected continuously over a long period before the policy's introduction and subsequent to it. The time of introducing the policy can be clearly identified, and regression models used to assess where the slope measuring change over time is different following the introduction of the policy compared to before the policy was introduced. One example is shown in Figure 8.1, panel A. The second example, shown in Figure 8.1, panel B, illustrates the 'difference-in-difference' method, where the control rate of change in an area without an intervention (grey line) is applied to an intervention region (dark line), and the dotted line shows how much change is expected to occur in that region ('x' amount of change). This can be compared when the actual change observed following the introduction of the intervention or policy from year 6 onwards ('y' amount of change) to indicate the difference that might be attributed to the intervention.

Inevitably, the greatest challenge in an NE over which the researcher has no control over exposure to the intervention is the strength of 'causal attribution': to what extent the evidence suggests that exposure to the event or policy caused the observed outcomes. Similar challenges arise in relation to external validity (generalisability), addressing the question of whether or not the same policy would have the same effects in a different region, country or context. As is the case with other evaluation designs and methodologies, understanding the differences between unexposed and exposed populations,

Figure 8.1 Examples of specialised evaluation designs commonly used in natural experiments

Panel A. Interrupted time series: year 4 new tobacco ban in Region A

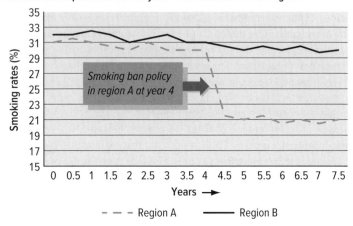

Panel B. Difference-in-difference analysis: NE policy introduction in year 6

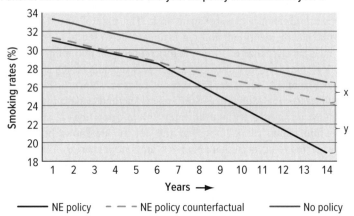

and the different ways in which demographic or other differences might explain observed outcomes, is equally challenging in the evaluation of NEs. Finally, it is important to recognise that NEs are separate from evaluations designed through researcher–policymaker partnerships; although these are sometimes described as NEs because there is some engagement of researchers in the design and methods used, they do not fit the definition provided above.

8.4 Summary

NEs are a new addition to program evaluation, especially for assessing the effects of health promotion and disease prevention policies. Given the strength of time-based (longitudinal) observations in NEs, and often a lack of competing explanations for the observed outcomes, the findings are often very useful to decision-makers and practitioners. NEs provide an innovative and additional suite of studies and methods to evaluate the population effects of events and policies to inform public health decisions.

References

Anyanwu PE, Craig P, Katikireddi SV, et al. (2020). Impact of UK tobacco control policies on inequalities in youth smoking uptake: a natural experiment study. Nicotine and Tobacco Research 22(11):1973–80.

Craig P, Cooper C, Gunnell D, et al. (2012). Using natural experiments to evaluate population health interventions: new Medical Research Council guidance. Journal of Epidemiology and Community Health 66(12):1182–6.

Craig P, Katikireddi SV, Leyland A, et al. (2017). Natural experiments: an overview of methods, approaches, and contributions to public health intervention research. Annual Review of Public Health 38:39–56.

Ejlerskov KT, Sharp SJ, Stead M, et al. (2018). Supermarket policies on less-healthy food at checkouts: natural experimental evaluation using interrupted time series analyses of purchases. PLoS Medicine 18 December;15(12):e1002712.

Fuller D, Luan H, Buote R, et al. (2019). Impact of a public transit strike on public bicycle share use: an interrupted time series natural experiment study. Journal of Transport & Health 13:137–42.

Islam N, Sharp SJ, Chowell G, et al. (2020). Physical distancing interventions and incidence of coronavirus disease 2019: natural experiment in 149 countries. BMJ 370:m2743.

Liyanage P, Rocklöv J, Tissera HA (2021). The impact of COVID-19 lockdown on dengue transmission in Sri Lanka: a natural experiment for understanding the influence of human mobility. PLoS Neglected Tropical Diseases 15(6):e0009420.

Moore G, Brown R, Page N, et al. (2020). Young people's use of e-cigarettes in Wales, England and Scotland before and after introduction of EU Tobacco Products Directive regulations: a mixed-method natural experimental evaluation. International Journal of Drug Policy 1 November;85:102795.

Sato K, Amemiya A, Haseda M, et al. (2020). Postdisaster changes in social capital and mental health: a natural experiment from the 2016 Kumamoto earthquake. American Journal of Epidemiology 189(9):910–21.

Scottish Government (n.d.). Social Research Group social science methods series. Guide 3: Natural Experiments. Accessed April 2022. https://tinyurl.com/2p94nm65

Further reading

Ogilvie D, Bauman A, Foley L, et al. (2020). Making sense of the evidence in population health intervention research: building a dry stone wall. BMJ Global Health 5(12):e004017.

9

Evidence, practice, policy and the critical practitioner

This chapter summarises some of the issues that impede or facilitate research translation and application in health promotion and prevention. As a part of this analysis we also consider necessary skills for the critical appraisal of evidence, enabling practitioners to make good decisions based on the strength and usefulness of published evidence.

9.1 Getting evidence into practice

Improving the quality and effectiveness of health promotion interventions ultimately depends on our ability to optimally use the evidence generated through research and evaluation. The central purpose of evaluation is to guide improvements in practice through the adoption of interventions that have a known and quantifiable impact on health and quality of life.

The use of evidence to guide decision-making in health promotion varies considerably and there are several reasons why this will be the case. In some circumstances sufficient 'evidence' of effectiveness does not exist or the evidence available may be insufficient to reach a conclusion in a timely way. For example, when a new public health threat emerges (such as COVID-19), rapid public health responses were needed in advance of the optimal level of evidence from careful research. In other cases where new public health challenges (such as e-cigarette use) emerge, there may be disagreement on the best mix of interventions to address the problem on a population basis (advocacy, education, social media campaigns, regulation and so on). For policymakers and practitioners, doing nothing in the absence of conclusive evidence is often not an option in the face of a public health emergency or community pressure for action.

When lacking clear evidence of effectiveness, those responsible for taking action (policymakers and practitioners) have to locate and prioritise the best available evidence from existing relevant studies and on information from practitioners and consumers. Responses have to be practical to implement and have potential for high population reach. Where an intervention has been initiated with limited relevant evidence, the case for evaluation is strong.

This not only allows for immediate learning from an experimental intervention (and enables adjustment to the intervention as it is implemented) but is also important for public accountability.

A model to illustrate differences in the use of evidence in health promotion programs is provided in Figure 9.1. One stage does not lead to another, but there is a proposed hierarchy that suggests better practice will be informed by theory and research evidence.

The *planned* approach is exemplified by the use of planning frameworks and logic models, as described in Chapters 1 and 2. This approach is based on rational, systematic assessment of the best available evidence of population health needs, effective interventions and the organisational and administrative conditions needed for successful intervention. This type of planning model represents the best evidence-based approach in health promotion, and links planning and evaluation in a logical sequence. Perceived community needs and the conditions necessary for the successful implementation of programs are accounted for in the planning process and through consultation during formative evaluation studies.

The *responsive* approach reflects a common situation for health promotion practitioners. It is typified by a high value on the role of a community in

Figure 9.1 Variation in the use of evidence in health promotion: planned, responsive and reactive practice (adapted from Nutbeam 1996)

Practice type	Features	
Planned	Systematic appraisal of evidence	
	Application of evidence according to sequential model	
	Higher level of practitioner control over decisions	Increasing use of research evidence
Responsive	Emphasis on responding to expressed need of target population	
	Commitment to partnership in control over decisions	
Reactive	Typically short-term, rapid response to perceived problems and crises	
	High level of central (government) control	

defining their health priorities and participating in the solution. In this case the *response* is to the perceived needs of an identified population. This approach which is characterised by co-development of programs is more likely to have the community participate in the intervention and to sustain its effects. But there are potential opportunity costs associated with responding to perceived community needs without sufficient consideration of the nature of the problems identified, or the evidence available about effective interventions.

Reactive practice is epitomised by short-term responses to a perceived problem or to a real (or perceived) public health crisis. Typically, resources are facilitated rapidly through a government agency for an urgent and usually high-profile response. Often this practice does not allow for an evidence-based response or significant community consultation. Success might be seen in terms of a high level of message penetration, and in some cases the relief of political pressure. Examples include public education campaigns that require an acute response, such as communications about COVID-19 prevention practices or environmental threats to health (e.g. an acute chemical pollution event or a heatwave). Regrettably, reactive practice may also reflect a more overtly political response to a public health problem, designed 'to be seen to act'; some anti-drug campaigns can be viewed in this light.

Although Figure 9.1 suggests a hierarchy of practice that places highest value on research evidence generated through a rational planning model, practitioners sometimes prefer a wider set of criteria to decide on priorities and intervention options. Practitioners who only adopt a highly structured approach to program planning may find themselves less able to respond to expressed community needs (a rewarding way to work) and political imperatives (a pragmatic way to work).

One of the frustrations facing diligent practitioners (and policymakers) is the paucity of relevant evaluation studies in the general literature on public health and health promotion. In reviewing the literature on any given topic, much is written that describes or helps to understand the problem, but there is limited intervention research to inform practical population-level responses. Further, many evaluations of interventions that are described as 'efficacious' are carried out in small, selected samples of people who participate in the research. Seldom do journals publish negative findings or suggest that interventions should be discontinued, although this would be of considerable benefit to decision-makers.

Research on health inequalities provides a good example of this frustration. In tackling health inequalities, there is often an inverse relationship between the volume and quality of available research, and the potential effectiveness of the interventions researched. For example, many interventions describe studies that modify individual behavioural risk. This research has often been conducted with small samples of people that are not representative of the social groups that need to be reached to reduce health inequalities, providing what some commentators have seen as the 'right answer to the wrong question'. By contrast, there is little intervention research that addresses some of the complex social, economic and environmental determinants of health. In terms of evaluation, this applies to comprehensive programs and scaled-up programs, where there is some description of process evaluation in the literature, but very few examples of outcomes achieved. Further, there is limited evidence of any kind to examine the relative costs and benefits of different intervention options.

It follows that research evidence can be more relevant for practice if researchers and funding agencies appreciate and fund more practice-relevant research, and especially evaluations of more comprehensive and complex interventions. Some practice-relevant evidence can be gathered instead from existing programs, by observing how they operate, identifying what has worked in the past and what has not, and learning from the experience of practitioners in delivering programs.

Evidence gathered from investigations of these types is often presented in the form of case studies, reflecting 'expert opinion' or even relatively anecdotal evidence. Such 'evidence' generally ranks much lower in established hierarchies of evidence but both practitioners and policymakers value it, particularly as it is often available when needed, and offers highly practical solutions that can be implemented.

In real-life circumstances, practitioners should seek a balance between conventional evidence of efficacy and effectiveness, and the flexibility of response that is required for population-level practice. Unsurprisingly, in this book we advocate a planned approach to health promotion practice, but we also recognise that in real-life circumstances, pragmatic adaptations are often needed.

9.2 Getting evidence into policy

Research evidence is used in different ways by policymakers. Research can have a direct role in framing policy, or in leading directly to policy change. However, it is not unusual that research evidence forms only one part of a complex and politicised process of policy decision-making. Evidence can be used selectively to justify predetermined positions that are largely ideologically driven. Though there are obvious exceptions, neither extremity in this range is sustainable.

Most policy change is incremental and based on a mix of influences. When opportunities for policy reform open up, policymakers will seek out the available evidence, but policy change is often constrained by established structures, investments and interests, and for these reasons is inherently political in nature. In this context, evidence is most often used if it fits within current policy priorities, and points to practical affordable actions. Disappointingly, in health promotion we too frequently fail one or more of these tests.

Regrettably, it is too often the case that the research questions of greatest interest to health promotion practitioners and to policymakers are not the questions that researchers are funded to answer. This means that decision-makers and practitioners may find it difficult to identify program evaluation information that is really useful to them. Solutions to this impasse have to come from dialogue between researchers, practitioners and policymakers to achieve greater practice relevance. In most countries, changes are needed to research funding processes to focus on achieving population-level change rather than small-scale individual change.

Much has been achieved in the development of methods for building, appraising and synthesising evidence, but it remains risky to consider evidence as 'sufficient' from only one study. The best policy-relevant evidence is where several studies across different settings generate consistent, similar findings. It is necessary to bridge the 'gap' between research evidence and the complexities of policy and practice using the methods of research translation (see Chapter 7). Resources should be prioritised to test promising ideas in different contexts, rather than to improve the effect sizes through minor variations to small-scale efficacy trials.

> *Working out which components work and which can be translated across different settings and social groups are of great importance to achieve population health gain.*

9.3 Critical appraisal of research and evaluation evidence

A major purpose of *Evaluation in a Nutshell* is to equip the reader with the ability to understand, interpret and assess the quality of published work in evaluation reports and in scientific journal papers. The preceding chapters have provided an introduction to many of the strategic and technical issues that arise in designing and conducting an evaluation. Understanding these principles will help in making judgments about the quality, relevance and applicability of 'evidence' described in the published research literature.

This ability to critically appraise published evidence is an important skill for all practitioners, researchers and decision-makers. *Critical appraisal* in health promotion requires a broad approach to judging the worth of interventions; this may need a conscious trade-off between the quality of evidence (as assessed by scientific and methodological rigour) and the practicality for implementation (often a question of judgment on a program's applicability to local circumstances).

The Appendix provides a critical appraisal checklist through which the health promotion relevance as well as the methodological rigour of a published study can be appraised (adapted from Bauman & Rissel 2003). Building on the key messages from each of the previous chapters, the checklist summarises the quality criteria for assessing formative, process and impact evaluation.

It is obvious that there is no single 'correct' answer for all forms of evaluation. For example, in a local pilot program, emphasis might be placed on formative and process evaluation. For judging excellence in effectiveness and efficacy studies, the standard criteria for assessing 'scientific' quality are used—evaluation design, measurement, sample size and appropriate approaches to the analyses of the results—but the relevance to local contexts and potential for whole population reach should also be considered. In scaling-up, we should always consider good process evaluation first, especially issues such as reach, context and program adaptations required in specific contexts.

This checklist could be used for reading any published evaluation in a peer-reviewed journal. Starting with the problem definition, Part A of the checklist includes careful documentation of the elements of formative and process evaluation (steps 2 and 3 in the Appendix), as well as describing and assessing the quality of scientific research methods used. By the time the discussion of the published paper is reached, it should be possible to assess the practice-based relevance and generalisability of the findings for your local circumstances and settings.

Criteria for the later phases of evaluation are shown in Part B of the checklist (steps 6 to 8 in the Appendix). For example, you might be searching for evidence of scaled-up efforts before considering the local adoption of a program. This search may include the *grey literature,* which comprises less-formal evaluations, published as technical monographs or evaluation reports from public sector or not-for-profit agencies. These may sometimes offer useful insight into the practical issues of implementation for practice.

Finally, thinking beyond the checklist, we need guidelines for summarising the quality of different types of evidence reviews that are available for a defined content area. These summaries use systematic research techniques to compare results from several interventions in a defined area, and answer specific questions on their usual effects. There are databases in which summaries are located, including the Cochrane Public Health Group, for assessing health promotion interventions. If outcomes and research designs are very similar, then a quantitative pooled analysis can summarise the net effects of a particular kind of intervention; this is known as a *meta-analysis*. In health promotion this is less frequent than in clinical and biomedical research, but examples relevant to health promotion and a link to relevant online repositories of evidence are on the companion Evaluation website: https://evaluationinanutshell.com/.

> *The ability to find evidence by accessing relevant reported research, and the ability to critically appraise evidence, are core skills in health promotion.*

9.4 Concluding comments: evaluation—art and science

A major purpose of *Evaluation in a Nutshell* is to provide an introduction to technical issues and challenges in the evaluation of health promotion programs. It becomes apparent that evaluating a health promotion program is both an art and a science.

The challenges we face stem from the diverse origins, goals and methods of health promotion programs. Evaluation should be integrated into a program plan from the beginning of a program idea (and the formative research that supports it), through to widespread program scale-up that should lead to population health change. Different evaluation designs and research methods are required for the different stages of program development, implementation and dissemination.

The various needs of researchers and practitioners result in the use of a range of qualitative and quantitative methods, producing 'evidence' for different purposes. Given this diversity, each project needs to consider the extent, expenditure and methodological rigour required for its evaluation, with the most appropriate methods used for the circumstances of the intervention. There is no single, correct evaluation design. Both qualitative and quantitative methods have an important place; both can be done well and both done badly, and one is not superior to the other.

For every health promotion intervention, careful formative and process evaluations are essential. Good planning will ensure that a quality program is developed; careful monitoring of implementation will contribute to an understanding of why one program works and another does not. Process evaluation is often neglected but it provides complementary information to program effectiveness, and is the cornerstone of the evaluation of replication and scaled-up programs.

To evaluate the effectiveness of a program, especially new programs, controlled or quasi-experimental research designs are essential. Established, reliable and valid impact measures should be used. The results should be assessed in terms of the observed *effect size*. Both qualitative and quantitative methods have an important place and, together, they can provide different perspectives on the effectiveness, feasibility and acceptability of interventions.

Recent developments in evaluating health promotion have influenced this book. The need to achieve population health outcomes means that practitioners and policymakers need to consider the complex 'systems' in which health is created, and this leads to new methods for comprehensive program evaluation. Mixed methods are more frequently used, and decisions need to be made about which components are the priority for evaluation. These decisions, and other aspects of evaluation planning and design, should be 'co-created' in partnerships between researchers, stakeholders and the community. Preparing for and evaluating programs at scale is important, with a focus on good process evaluation to assess reach and adaptation; without these process attributes being successful, sustainable population health improvement will not occur.

Ultimately, not all of us have the opportunity or resources to undertake highly structured evaluation of our work. Better knowledge of the strategic and technical issues in health promotion evaluation enables us to make well-informed judgments of published work and also to evaluate our own work as *critical practitioners*. This knowledge is of great importance in managing the expectations of managers, funders and the wider community.

References

Bauman A & Rissel C (2003). Guidelines for journal reviewing. Health Promotion Journal of Australia 4(2):79–82.

Nutbeam D (1996). Achieving 'best practice' in health promotion: improving the fit between research and practice. Health Education Research 11(3):317–26.

appendix

Critical appraisal checklist for health promotion programs

This appendix has been adapted and updated from Bauman A & Rissel C (2003). Guidelines for journal reviewing. Health Promotion Journal of Australia 4(2):79–82.

Part A: Appraisal of individual interventions

1. Problem definition

- Is the health problem a public health priority? Is it a government or policy priority?
- What is the magnitude of the problem, and which population subgroups are at higher risk?

2. Formative evaluation and program development

- Is the problem amenable to change, through a feasible intervention? Does a literature search identify effective interventions? If there are several published studies, are there summaries of the evidence (non-systematic or systematic reviews); or formal pooled estimates from multiple studies (using statistical techniques of meta-analysis)? From this review, what effect size is generally observed for this intervention?
- Is there evidence of piloting or testing of the intervention or its component parts?
- Was the intervention tested with people similar to the proposed target group?
- Was there an underlying theoretical framework or conceptual model for the intervention?
- Were the intervention strategies and settings identified as 'best practice' (evidence-based) approaches?

■ Are there funds for the intervention to be delivered as planned, and is there sufficient time for expected effects or changes to be observed?

■ Was there a logic model to describe the ways that the intervention/ program might work? (This will inform the priorities for which components warrant evaluation.)

3. Process evaluation

■ Is there evidence of process evaluation to monitor the implementation, reach and participant acceptance of the program or its components?

■ Is there evidence of adaptation of the intervention, fitting the intervention into different settings (and whether the effects were similar in different contexts)?

■ How many people received (attended, participated in) the intervention? Were they typical of the target group (or were they different to those who did not participate)? Of all those who could participate or be included, how many actually did so?

4. Research methods to appraise the stages of impact and outcome evaluation

Study (research) design

■ What was the study (research) design in this evaluation? Was it the most feasible study design that might have been used in this setting within available resources? Will the design provide sufficient rigour to demonstrate good-quality evidence of effectiveness?

Study sample

■ What is the target population? Are the people who actually participated in the intervention typical of the target population? Were there any selection effects (e.g. non-representative/volunteer participants) that might influence the conclusions on program effectiveness?

■ How were people recruited into, or how did they volunteer for, the study?

Measurement

■ Are there specified and measurable intervention objectives?

■ Are all relevant processes and outcomes assessed? How important are any omitted outcomes?

■ Were the measuring tools, questionnaire or instruments reliable and valid?

■ Were qualitative methods and measures used appropriately to explain how and why the program worked?

Analysis

- Was the sample size of participants assessed in the evaluation sufficient to detect any potential effects (sufficient statistical power)?
- Were there any factors that were not measured that might have influenced the findings? Were these factors able to be controlled for in the analysis?
- Were the most appropriate approaches to quantitative and qualitative analyses used?

General

- Was the time frame for proposed changes clearly stated? Is it realistic? Does the evaluation clearly measure all relevant changes (outcomes)?
- Was there any other corroborating evidence to support or refute the observed effects (either from changes in other outcomes or from qualitative evaluation data)?
- [Specifically for comprehensive program evaluations (CPEs)] Was there evidence of an integrated set of planning and implementation tasks? Were all components evaluated using appropriate methods (quantitative and qualitative)?

5. Interpretation/discussion of the results

- Were the conclusions drawn by the author(s) justified by their data?
- Were the findings generalisable to the whole community or to similar populations/settings?
- Were any reported significant effects of practical health promotion significance or were they simply of statistical significance?
- Did the formative or process evaluation components of the evaluation enable us to understand how or why the health promotion program worked? Especially for negative studies, might additional information have been informative here?
- Is there a need for replication research in this area; or, if the intervention appeared to be ineffective, what alternative approaches might be developed to address this problem?

Part B: Post-intervention appraisal—making a public health difference?

6. Replication and scale-up

- Was planning for scale-up considered in the initial efficacy/ effectiveness intervention?

- Has the initial effective/efficacious intervention subsequently been implemented and tested in a range of more representative settings (generalisability)?
- Were the programs implemented and delivered successfully (mostly adhering to program objectives and methods) in different settings; or, if implementation differed, what difference did adaptation make to outcomes observed?
- Were effective intervention results communicated to policymakers and to professionals and practitioners? Is there a defined advocacy strategy to scale-up this program? (This is knowledge translation—see Rychetnik et al. [2012].)

7. Scale-up (dissemination)

- What mechanisms for scale-up are possible and affordable?
- Is there a 'policy window' (Lee et al. 2020) when governments, non-government organisations or the private sector might provide support and resources to deliver the program at a population scale?

8. Institutionalisation

- Are there policy changes in place to support and resource the sustainment and institutionalisation of the effective program?
- Are there quality assurance systems in place to monitor program sustainability and assess the delivery and fidelity of program components (process evaluation)?
- Are there surveillance systems to monitor the impact/outcomes of interest at the population level (e.g. improvements in physical activity levels; increased immunisation rates; increased cancer screening uptake)?

References

Lee K, van Nassau F, Grunseit A, et al. (2020). Scaling up population health interventions from decision to sustainability—a window of opportunity? A qualitative view from policymakers. Health Research Policy and Systems Dec;18(1):1–2.

Rychetnik L, Bauman A, Laws R, et al. (2012). Translating research for evidence-based public health: key concepts and future directions. Journal of Epidemiology and Community Health 66(12):1187–92.

Glossary*

Advocacy A combination of individual and social actions designed to gain political commitment, policy support, social acceptance and systems support for a particular health goal or program.

Behavioural epidemiology The study of the distribution (how much of a problem in the population) and determinants of (causal factors that lead to) behaviours that are related to health (see p. 25).

Bias Where something differs systematically from the true situation. Biases found in studies may be due to how people are selected, how they choose to volunteer for a program (*selection bias;* see Box 5.1, p. 65) or how they are assessed or measured (*measurement or information bias;* see Box 5.2, pp. 69–71).

Causality Scientific evidence that the intervention or program 'caused' any changes observed in outcomes.

Cluster randomised control trial A randomised controlled trial (RCT) where randomisation occurs at the level of groups or communities (see pp. 59–60). See also **randomised controlled trial (RCT).**

Cohort An identified group or population. In a cohort study, the same population is followed and assessed at each stage in the study, both before and after an intervention. Cohorts are sometimes used in **quasi-experimental design** studies.

Comprehensive program evaluation (CPE) The process of designing and conducting evaluations of complex (public health) programs. These are multi-component interventions targeting multi-faceted problems in whole populations or community settings and using a diverse range of strategies to influence any or all of individuals, settings, professionals or policymakers.

Confidence interval (or *confidence limits*) Statistical terms that describe whether the observed result in a study is outside of a range of possible results within which the true value in the population is likely to lie.

Consultation The process of engaging with or seeking the views of stakeholders, the community or target group members, with a view to enabling participation and *co-creation* in intervention development, advocacy or policy formulation. See also **participatory planning.**

Contamination The amount to which control or comparison groups or communities might be exposed to intervention elements (see pp. 59–60).

Content validity See **validity.**

Correlate(s) Factors that are statistically associated with other variables. Correlation does not imply causality.

Cross-sectional study A survey, or other form of data collection, that is obtained at a single point in time from a population or population sample. Unlike a **cohort** study, these individuals are not followed and assessed on a further occasion.

---

*The definitions in this glossary are pragmatic definitions based on the authors' experiences in evaluation, research and practice in health promotion. Where detailed definitions are provided earlier in the book, the chapters/pages are referred to here. More formal definitions can be found in publications such as:
- Porta M (ed.) (2014). A Dictionary of Epidemiology. Oxford University Press.
- Nutbeam D & Muscat DM (2021). Health promotion glossary 2021. Health Promotion International Dec;36(6):1578–98.

Dissemination An active and intentional process of scaling-up an intervention to maximise uptake and impact in a community.

Drop out or loss to follow up The proportion of participants who start a program or are included in a study, and do not participate in follow-up activities or surveys—they are 'lost to follow up'. This may lead to **bias** in the results if those individuals who maintain participation are systematically different from those who drop out. See also **non-response bias.**

Effectiveness The extent to which an intervention or program is successful in 'real-life' conditions in achieving the impact and outcomes that were predicted during the planning of the program.

Effect size A quantitative metric that describes the size of the difference in effectiveness between intervention and control groups in a standardised way that can be compared among studies.

Efficacy The extent to which a health promotion intervention is successful (in achieving its proposed outcomes) under controlled or 'best possible' conditions; usually characterised by optimal scientific designs.

Evaluation The process of judging the value of something. In health promotion, an evaluation will determine the extent to which a program has achieved its desired outcomes, and will assess the different processes that led to these outcomes. See also **formative evaluation, process evaluation** and **impact evaluation.**

Evaluation design The set of procedures and tasks that need to be carried out to examine the implementation, impact and outcomes of a health promotion intervention. Also sometimes referred to as *research design* or *study design,* which usually refers to the designs of the quantitative evaluation of program effectiveness or efficacy.

Fidelity (or *program fidelity*) The part of **process evaluation** that examines whether or not the intervention/program was delivered using the methods and materials as designed and intended with the proposed target audiences.

Formative evaluation A set of activities designed to develop, identify and test program materials and methods. Formative evaluation usually occurs as part of program planning and occurs before any elements of the program are implemented.

Generalisability (or *external validity*) The extent to which the findings from the study are likely to be reproduced in other groups or in the whole population.

Health outcomes The long-term endpoints of a health promotion program. They may include reduced morbidity and mortality, improved quality of life and functional independence.

Health promotion outcomes Modifiable personal, social and environmental factors that are a means of changing the determinants of health (**intermediate health outcomes**). They also represent the more immediate results of planned health promotion activities.

Impact evaluation A set of activities designed to assess short-term effects or efficacy of an intervention. This may include measurement of health promotion and intermediate health outcomes.

Institutionalisation Where a program has been successfully scaled-up across a community, has established policy support and funding mechanisms and has continuing community support. This stage of evaluation is primarily concerned with quality control and long-term monitoring and surveillance of outcomes at a population level.

Intermediate health outcomes The results of health promotion programs in the short term, which are measured by changes in lifestyle factors (e.g. food choices, physical activity, substance use), accessing preventive services or environment changes that are likely to lead to improved health outcomes.

Level of measurement A way of describing **variables** in a study. Levels of measurement include: continuous (interval) data, such as height or blood pressure; ranked data that has ordered categories, such as from 'like a lot' through to 'do not like at all'; and categorical (discrete) data which has a range of named categories by which the data can be described (such as occupational group, gender or language spoken). Sometimes the data has only two categories (yes/no, smoker/non-smoker), which are described as 'dichotomous' or 'binary' variables. See **measures and indicators**.

Logic model A way of describing the changes that the program is intended to bring about, defining what will happen during a program, in what order and with what anticipated effects (see Box 1.1, p. 13). This is a conceptual 'roadmap' that reflects how a program will be planned and implemented, and describe the intended effects. A logic model is similar to *intervention mapping.*

Measures and indicators Both assess and measure objects of interest (behaviours, knowledge, participation). 'Measures' are usually related to **impact** and **outcome evaluation** and are central to demonstrating efficacy/effectiveness of programs. 'Indicators' are often **process evaluation** measures, such as quality measures, measures of services and measures of policy (see p. 69).

Meta-analysis This is a quantitative research synthesis through pooling data from different interventions to obtain an average assessment of effectiveness across studies.

Non-observable phenomena Attributes or characteristics (such as knowledge, attitudes, public opinion and even some health behaviours) that cannot be directly observed and have to be indirectly measured (e.g. through validated surveys or interviews). This is different to *observable phenomena,* such as a diagnosed health condition or body weight.

Non-response bias The differences in the variables of interest in a study between those participating or completing a study (or intervention program) and those who do not participate.

Objectives Health promotion program objectives are measurable changes to modifiable personal attributes (such as knowledge, motivations and skills), social norms and social support, and organisational factors (e.g. rules and processes) that influence the program goals. See also **health promotion outcomes.**

Outcome evaluation A set of activities designed to assess whether or not the program successfully achieved its *endpoint goals* (such as changes in health behaviours) and *intermediate objectives* (such as improved knowledge and skills). Usually, outcomes imply longer term changes such as health status, whereas shorter term endpoints are often described as program impact. See also **impact evaluation.**

Participatory planning A process of engaging with communities or stakeholders to form partnerships. These partnerships result in *co-creation* of a program, where the planning process is carried out through consultations and community forums to make decisions about the content or delivery of programs that may improve health.

Pilot testing A set of activities designed to assess the feasibility and/or relevance of intervention components (see **formative evaluation**). Pilot testing may also refer to measurement development and piloting of a measurement in a sample of people. This is used to assess the **reliability** and **validity** of a proposed measurement.

Pre–post study A one-group evaluation design (also known as a 'before–after study'). This is in the category of pre-experimental study designs. This can be a relatively weak design with a single group measured before and after an intervention. This design is often used in pilot studies to estimate the likely effect of an intervention.

Prevalence A measure that describes the proportion of people who are affected by, or have a particular condition, in a defined population.

Process evaluation A set of activities designed to assess the success and factors surrounding program implementation. Process evaluation describes and explains what happens once the program has actually started, and the extent to which the program is implemented and delivered as planned (see **fidelity**).

Program plan Usually a written document that specifies the interventions to be employed, the sequence of activities, the partnerships to be developed, the personnel to be involved at different stages and the costs of the interventions. See also **logic model.**

Project or intervention (compared to a **program of work**; see Table 1.1, p. 1). A discrete project or intervention is usually based on the use of a single method or single intervention strategy in a clearly defined setting; a more comprehensive program of work, using multiple intervention/project strategies in different settings and targeting multiple groups, requires more complex program evaluation (see **comprehensive program evaluation** and Chapter 6).

Qualitative methods Descriptive and analytical research techniques that are used to explore and explain phenomena of interest. Methods include the use of focus groups (structured discussions with stakeholders or members of a target group) or directly learning from participating in or with target group members (ethnographic research or participant observation, sometimes called 'action research').

Quantitative methods Descriptive and analytical research techniques that

are intended to produce numeric data amenable to statistical analysis. Such data allows statistical testing of comparisons between groups, trends over time or the strength of associations between variables.

Quasi-experimental designs Evaluation designs that have defined control or comparison populations against which intervention group effects could be compared. The population or group receiving the intervention is predetermined and non-randomly assigned; a pre–post design may be classified as a quasi-experimental design if there are multiple time points of observation (one-group **time series;** see p. 61).

Random sample A sample drawn from a population where each individual has an equal probability of being chosen. Random sampling is intended to produce a sample that is **representative** of the population.

Randomised controlled trial (RCT) A research design where the individuals (or groups) receiving the intervention are randomly allocated to receive the program (*intervention* or *experimental* group) or not to receive the program (*control* or *comparison* group). Every individual or group has an equal chance of being offered the program. If allocation is at the group or institutional level, it is called a **cluster randomised controlled trial** (see pp. 59–60).

Reach A term used to describe the proportion of a target population that is engaged in the elements of an intervention or program. Reach is important in determining the generalisability of a program to a population as a whole. The concept of reach is also relevant to the **replication** and **scale-up (dissemination)** stages of program evaluation. See also **generalisability.**

Reliability The stability of a measure, assessing the extent to which each time the measure is used, and for each person it is used with, it will measure the same thing (give the same score or value). Reliability may also be assessed through two or more individuals assessing the same phenomenon; the level of agreement between them is referred to as *inter-rater reliability.*

Replication The process of repeating an effective intervention in a different setting or with a different population or subgroup to assess whether intervention effects are similar or different.

Representativeness (Usually of data or information from a sample of people.) Sample representativeness describes how well the included or observed sample reflects the overall population of interest. If the results of an evaluation are from a representative sample, then the results will be more *generalisable.*

Responsiveness The capacity of a measurement for change in response to an intervention. The best responsive measures should show a substantial change following an intervention, but not show change in the absence of an intervention.

Sample A group of individuals selected from a population for study or to be participants in a health promotion intervention. Special types of samples are described on page 65. See also **random sample.**

Sample size calculation How many people are needed for an evaluation study using standard statistical formulas. To do this, it is necessary to specify what quantitative change is expected or hoped for in the intervention (e.g. a 10% increase in breast cancer screening from 70% to 80% following the intervention).

Scales or scores Composite summaries of existing **variables** intended to produce an overall score to reflect an underlying dimension (e.g. six questions—or items— might be summed to produce an overall 'depression score').

Scaling-up interventions Defined as an intervention previously efficacious/effective in a small-scale study or trial that has been expanded under real-world conditions to

reach a greater proportion of the eligible population. (See Chapter 7.)

Secular trends Describe the rate of background changes in a phenomenon over a long period of time in a population (e.g. national rates of smoking might be declining, and obesity rates may be increasing over time).

Statistical significance A measure of the extent to which the relationship between variables, or observed results, from a study might have occurred by chance. Statistical significance is assessed after the application of appropriate statistical tests.

Structured discussions A qualitative research method to elicit information or perceptions from structured questions that are defined in advance. Structured discussions may be with individuals, or with groups of people, such as focus groups.

Summative evaluation This is an overview term to describe the different levels of evaluation, process and impact, and can also include economic evaluation. Summative evaluation often involves **triangulation** of data to reach a conclusion about a program's overall usefulness and effectiveness.

System-wide program evaluation Integrates and incorporates the different elements in 'the system' into a comprehensive program evaluation. The system includes health services and delivery settings. The population system for health promotion is often broader, with multiple stakeholders, multiple agencies and multiple interventions. Evaluation needs to assess the workings of the system (partnerships, co-creation of programs), as well as usual process and impact/outcome evaluation.

Time-series design The set of procedures used to evaluate a health promotion intervention in which there are multiple measurements preceding intervention, followed by multiple post-intervention measurements of the outcome of interest.

Triangulation The process of comparing different evaluation findings that are accumulated from a variety of sources; for example, comparing results on program effectiveness by examining quantitative data, and then considering if qualitative information points to the same direction and degree of effectiveness.

Validity The assessment of the 'truth' of a measurement. A question, scale or score is considered valid to the extent it measures what it intended to measure. Types of validity include 'face validity', whether experts in the field think the measure is a useful way of assessing the dimension of interest, and 'content validity', the items that cover all of the potential areas ('domains') of interest. 'Construct validity' describes the extent to which the construct that is being measured in a study (e.g. self-efficacy, social capital or quality of life) is actually measured by the questions or items used in a study. The usual methods for identifying a construct is through statistical techniques that we are not able to cover in this book, such as latent variable methods, exploratory or confirmatory factor analysis, internal consistency reliability and structural equation modelling.

Variables Quantitative measures that are (validly and reliably) assessed and, as the name suggests, capable of showing variation between subjects, and variation in response to intervention. Variables may be single items (single questions) or summarised as composite **scales or scores.**

index

Page numbers in **bold** print refer to main entries.

A

academics, xiv
'action research,' 32
actions *see* health promotion actions
advocacy, 8, 9, 123
analysis of data, 32, **66-8,** 121, *see also* statistical tests
assessment of uptake, 97

B

before-after (pre-post) studies, 63, 94
behavioural epidemiology, 25, 123
best practice, identifying, 37-9
bias, 123
  non-response, 65
  response, 73
  selection, **64-6**

C

case studies
  formative evaluation, using, 40-42
  health promotion interventions, 28, 29-31
  immunisation, 31
  physical activity promotion, 25, 29
  skin cancer prevention, 28, 31
  stages of evaluation, 29-31
  sun protection, 28, 31, 85
causality, 123
cluster randomised controlled trials, 28, 61, 84, 123
cohort studies, 62, 73, 123
community
  consultation with target groups, 37, 39
  impact of program over time on, 10-11
  value judgments by, xiv
comparison groups, 60
comparison populations, 60, 62

comprehensive program evaluations (CPEs), 18, **78-89,** 123
  calculating cost-effectiveness, 87
  challenges in conducting, 85-7
  examples in published papers, 87-8
  formative evaluation, 82
  impact/outcome evaluation and research designs for, 83-4
  planning for, 80-85
  process evaluation for, 82-3
  summative evaluation, 84-5
concepts, 71
confidence intervals, 67, 123
confounding factors, 68
consistency in scales and scores, 71
construct validity, 71
consultation with target groups, 37, 123
contamination (of control groups), 60, 123
content validity, 71, 123
context, 49, 50, 83, 116
continuous measure, 67
control groups, 60
controlled trials, 58-62
control (comparison) populations, 60
  quasi-experimental designs, 62-4
convenient sampling, 65, 66
correlates of health outcomes, 25, 123
cost-effectiveness, calculating, 87
COVID-19, 41, 103
  immunisation program, 86
  prevention practices, 113
COVID-19 health promotion program, 7, 9-10
critical appraisal of evidence, **115-17**
critical practitioners, 111, **118**
cross-sectional studies, 62, 123
  response bias and, 73

D

data analysis, 32, **66-8,** 121, *see also* statistical tests
data collection, 31-3, 67, 80, 82, 84, 104